Towards a
POST-FLEXNERIAN REVOLUTION

Graduating the Virtuous Physician

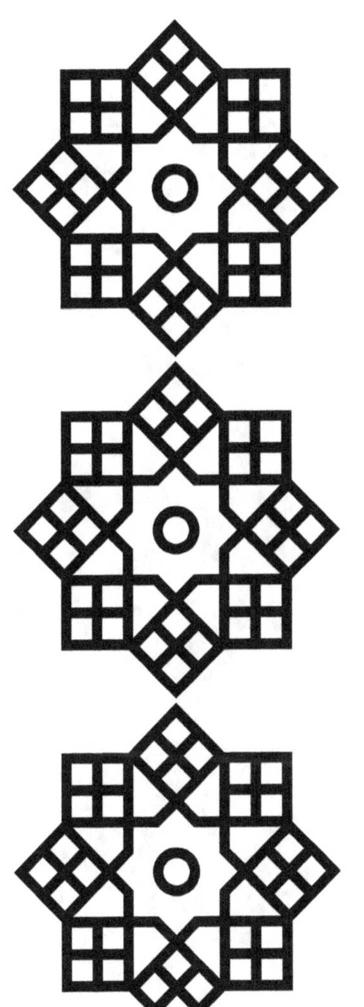

Towards a

POST-FLEXNERIAN REVOLUTION

Graduating the Virtuous Physician

Thalia Arawi

American University of Beirut Press

©2020 by the American University of Beirut

For requests and permissions, contact aubpress@aub.edu.lb

Printed in Beirut, Lebanon
ISBN 978-9953-586-41-0

CONTENTS

...to Mama, the light of my being
who raised me on virtues, morals,
and courage.

1.1. INTRODUCTION

In Plato's *The Republic*, Glaucon resorts to a thought experiment and introduces the legend of the ring of Gyges whereby a shepherd comes into possession of a ring that makes him invisible. Armed with this power, he starts to act unjustly. He seduces the queen, murders the king, and seizes the throne.[1] Fearless of reprisals, he demonstrates that even a just man might behave unjustly, rendering his actions unseen and unpunished. With this myth, Plato illustrated an important and eternal truth around which this book revolves: the good person will do the right thing regardless of punishment or reward.

Applied to the practice of medicine, one can argue that the same pertains to the fine physician. She will be the kind of physician who will do what is right even when there is no one to judge her. Several forces make this ideal difficult to reach, the same forces that attack what has come to be known as medical professionalism: market forces, personal corruption, the economic situation, to mention but a few. Nonetheless, it is my contention that although this ideal is difficult to achieve, it is not an impossibility, for idealism may be seen as another face of realism. One way to achieve it is by nurturing good and virtuous physicians who acknowledge that the profession of medicine will have to work by a new formula: $m=ec2$, namely, that medicine is about empathy, care, and cure.

This book attempts to address this issue, raising the following question: what can medical schools do in order to ensure that their graduates will possess a fine character? Put differently, what can medical schools do to graduate physicians who will serve the ends of medicine as a profession, not a trade, and who will *do the right thing even when no one is looking*? Although this book stresses the importance of virtues and their development in the neophyte physician, it is not a book on virtue ethics. Rather it is a work on the moral education of the neophyte physician. Throughout the book, I have assumed the general setting of the US educational system and in particular its use in Lebanon.

Chapter one presents a view of medicine as a moral endeavor based on a covenant of trust and argues that ethics and virtues are essential for the making of a fine physician. In this chapter, I discuss some of the basic ideas of Edmund Pellegrino about the ends of medicine being "internal" to the profession. Starting from this

---

1. Plato, *The Republic*, trans. Francis MacDonald Cornford (Oxford: Oxford University Press, 1942), 43–44.

assumption, it follows that medical schools need to educate students of medicine in ethics and virtues.

Chapter two begins by briefly presenting Aristotle's virtue ethics and the role that they can and perhaps should play in the moral development of medical students during their years of training in medical schools. Thus I argue that virtue ethics play an important role in the formation of the good neophyte physician who will eventually *do the right thing even when no one is looking*. I maintain that if virtue is to be taught, physicians in training need good role models, and medical schools need to provide an organizational structure and a culture that allow for the growth of virtues.

Chapter three tackles the main theme of education: If medical students are to be trained in the virtues, which curricular reforms would achieve this? Accordingly, this chapter begins by looking at the different types of curricula that play a role in the making of the future physician. It shows that the hidden curriculum is far too important to be neglected and, as such, plays a crucial role in ensuring that changes take place in the right direction and that moral erosion of future physicians will be avoided.[2]

Chapter four deals with the issue of whether medical schools, in addition to enacting curricular reform, can ensure that their graduates will actually do the right thing; that they will concern themselves with the "internal ends" of medicine. I argue that this can be done mostly by working with veteran physicians who will serve as role models and mentors in an appropriate institutional culture. Hence, this chapter offers suggestions that can be taken up by medical schools in the hope of being able to graduate virtuous physicians, recommending what I call a *post-Flexnerian revolution*.

To summarize, almost all medical schools offer their students clinical training that prepares them to become skilled medical practitioners. This book argues that medical schools need to do more than that. They should also offer their students character training that will equip them to become good medical doctors whose character will drive them to act virtuously, whether or not anyone is looking.

---

2. The hidden curriculum will be discussed further in chapter 3.

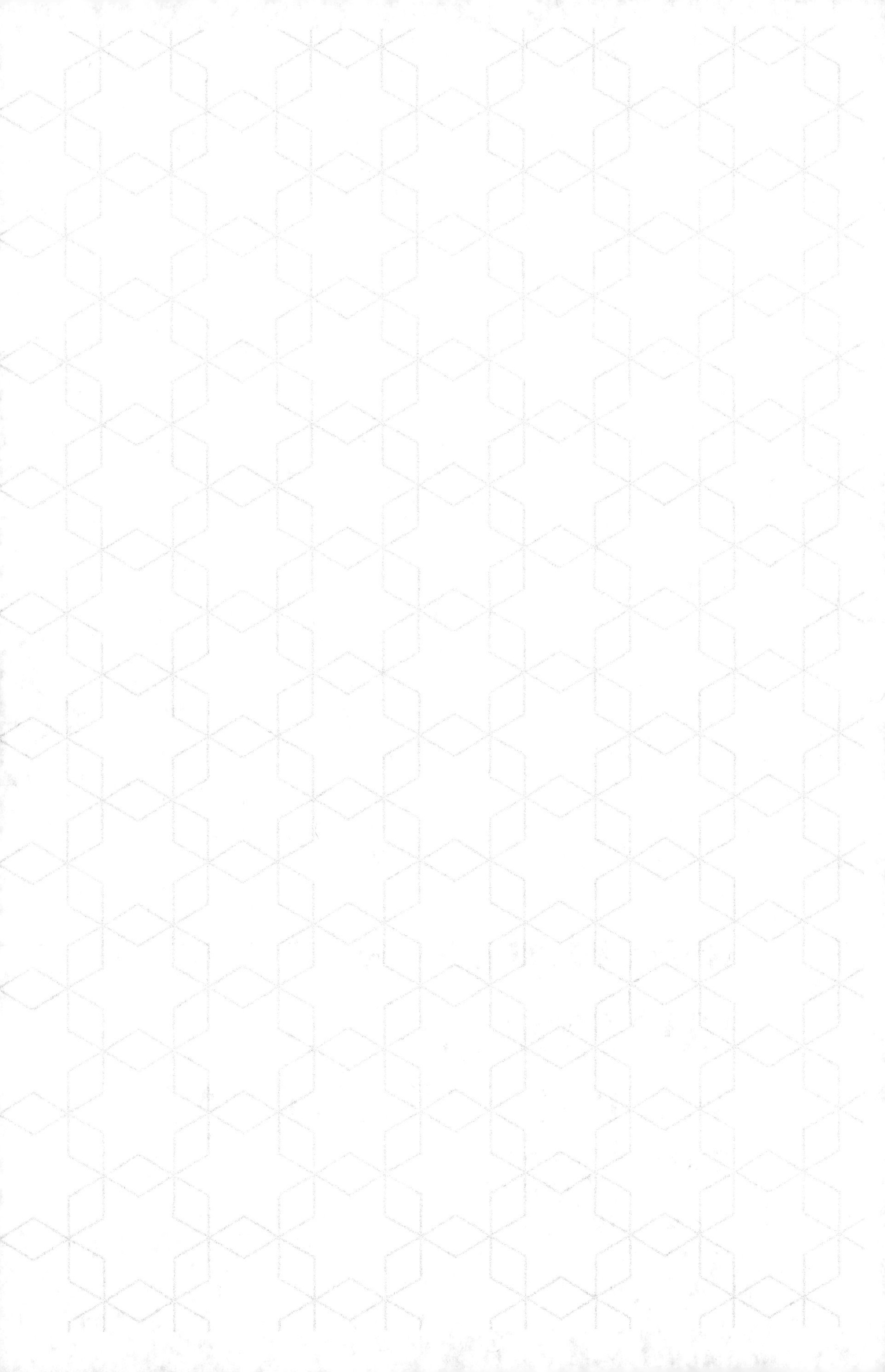

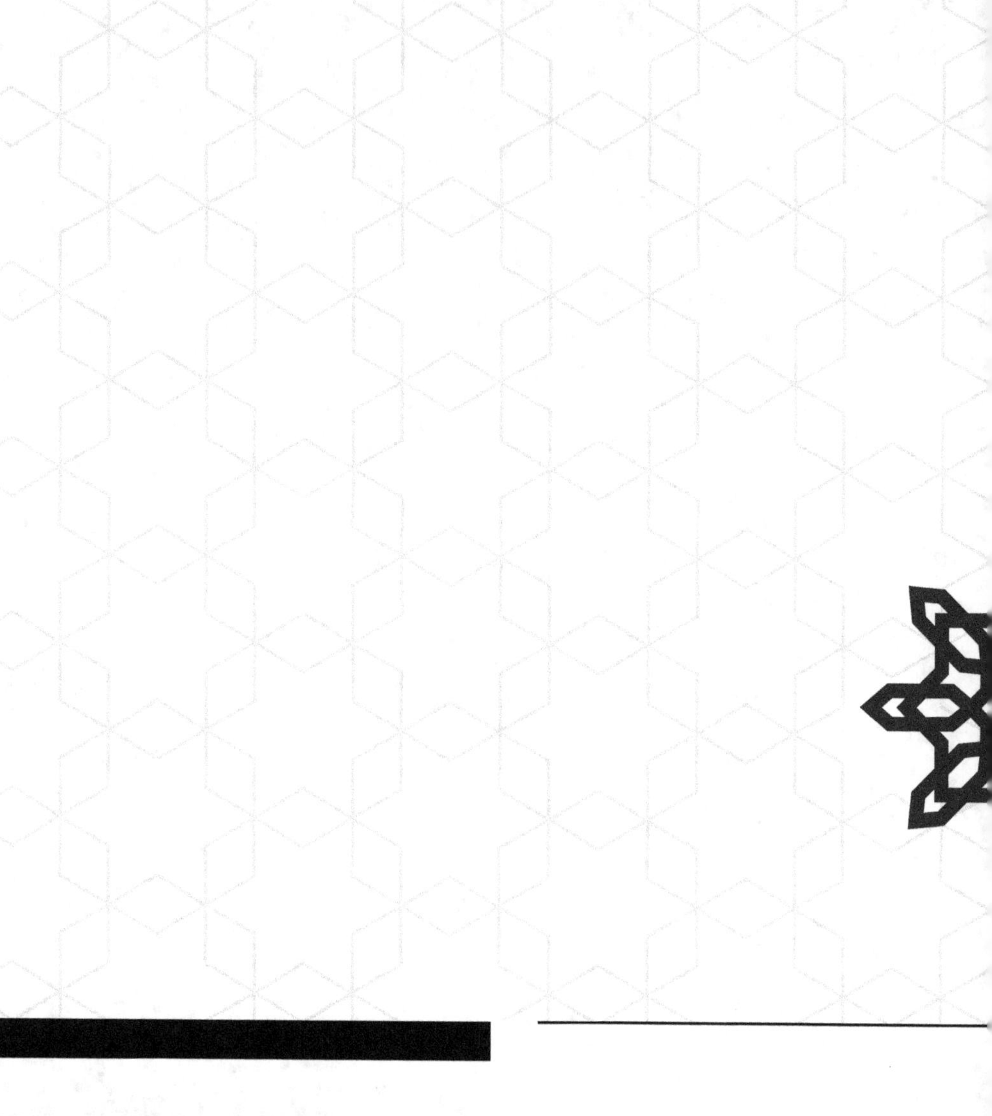

CHAPTER 1:
MEDICINE AS A MORAL ENDEAVOR

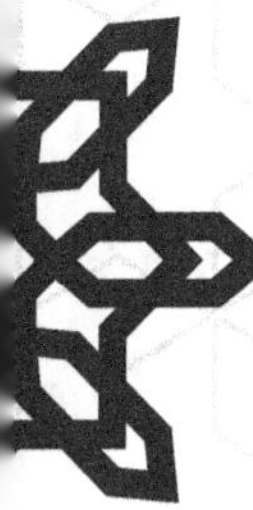

Every art and every inquiry, and similarly every action and pursuit, is thought to aim at some good; and for this reason the good has rightly been declared to be that at which all things aim.

—*Aristotle, Nicomachean Ethics (1947, 308)*

I n *The Death of Ivan Ilych*, Tolstoy recounts the story of a man living his last days, preoccupied with the thoughts that he has not lived the successful life he thought he ought to have lived, that most of his life has been a lie. At one point, Ivan falls sick and is advised to visit a famous physician, but the visit does not go well. At the end of the visit, Ivan, the patient, says nothing, but he ". . . rose, placed the doctor's fee on the table, and remarked with a sigh: 'We sick people probably often ask inappropriate questions. But tell me, in general, is this complaint dangerous, or not?'" (Tolstoy 1967, 271). The facts are that when the physician first met the patient, "he put on just the same air towards him as he himself put on towards an accused person" (1967, 270). He assumed an air of distance and indifference, and treated Ivan impersonally, as a disease or a number, while for Ivan this illness was something that affected his inner being. His experience of pain and mortality had shattered his being. Yet, the physician, though skilled and renowned, ignored that part of him—his inner being. Indeed, something in the physician was wanting. Precisely for this reason, Ivan could not be healed under his care. Ivan's physician-patient experience represented a clinical encounter that failed to provide what is needed for a good healing relationship. The patient was powerless in the face of a physician who was uncaring.

In this chapter, I argue that medicine is intrinsically a moral endeavor, and hence ethics and virtues are vital for the making of any physician, let alone a fine one.[1] It follows from this that medical schools need to educate students of medicine in ethics and virtues. Virtues must be internalized to become second nature to the medical student. This is how the "ends of medicine" will be met and the profession of medicine safeguarded. Assuming that medicine is a moral enterprise, I present the views of Edmund Pellegrino regarding the ends of medicine,[2] offering a critique of them whenever his arguments are inconsistent. I also discuss the importance of trust in the physician-patient relationship and argue that trust is a quintessential part of this relationship, which has been damaged in the course of modern-day medical practices. The development of good character in the physician is essential in order to salvage the clinical encounter from serious breakdown.

---

1. In this book, the terms "ethics" and "morals" are used interchangeably. It is my contention that a physician deserves to be called such only if she is ethical and follows the appropriate norms of her profession; otherwise, she is, at best, a qualified and skilled medical technician.

2. This concept will be expanded on later in this chapter.

1.1. Why Edmund Pellegrino?

Among the most prominent thinkers who have written about the ends of medicine are Howard Brody and Franklin G. Miller, and Robert M. Veatch. Yet, my decision to focus on the views of Edmund Pellegrino is precisely because, in addition to being a physician, he has spent a lifetime as a philosopher of medicine and his philosophy is based on reflections on years of practice. He has interacted with numerous patients and healthcare workers and has spent a considerable amount of time reflecting on the role of the healer from the perspective of a practicing physician. In doing so, he has managed to bridge the gap between theory and practice. Moreover, his concerns and research questions are the same ones I have often reflected on while considering what is happening in practice. For both of us, medicine is an art as well as a science, a moral enterprise that cannot be entirely isolated from the humanities. Ultimately, what is most needed to safeguard medicine from an impending downfall hastened by rapidly developing scientific technology is the commitment to the making of a humane physician; I largely share his views. Most importantly, while writing about what ought to be, Pellegrino starts from a reflection on the realities of medicine, arguing that we should be mindful of blind utopianism. Thus, one of the main strengths of his thinking lies in the fact that, unlike philosophers whose work is mainly theoretical, his ideas are actually based on real life practice. He has worked with suffering patients, held the stethoscope, felt the vulnerability and the anguish of patients, experienced the duties and the tensions, and reflected on all these matters. A philosopher who speculates and makes arguments, however strong, out of pure a priori analysis detached from the realities of everyday life cannot be more convincing than Pellegrino, whose philosophical reflections are grounded in what he has lived. I say this firmly because my work on the wards and my interactions with members of the healthcare teams as well as with patients and families have allowed me to see matters differently than I might have if the matter had been purely theoretical.

We live in times when we cannot afford speculation and incantations. We need reflections based on facts and empirical findings, and this is precisely what Pellegrino's reflections offer. More importantly, such thoughts are a requisite characteristic of medical ethics, a branch of practical ethics that distinguishes it from pure theoretical ethics and abstract philosophy. When asked, "How do you know?" Pellegrino's response is: "I've been there."

1.2. Medicine as a Moral Enterprise

Let me begin with a true story: Mrs. A was ready for a normal vaginal delivery and everything was progressing smoothly. The attending physician, the resident doctor, and a third-year medical student were gathered around the patient. Suddenly, the attending physician asked the nurse to get a pair of forceps and started explaining to the resident how a baby is delivered using that instrument. The student, sensitive to issues pertaining to ethics and the rights of patients, dared to ask the attending physician about the reason for resorting to a nonindicated forceps delivery. The reply was plain: the resident had never delivered by forceps and the attending physician wanted to teach him. This was, after all, a teaching hospital. Neither the mother nor the father had an idea of what was happening. After the procedure was over, the note on the medical chart indicated "normal vaginal delivery." One cannot but ponder whether medicine in such cases is seen as a purely scientific activity isolated from ethical issues.

In addition to the fact that both mother and newborn were exposed to medical risks that could have been avoided, several other ethical issues arise. The one that baffled the student most was that this obstetrician previously had lectured them about ethics and the importance of putting the interest of patients first. Looking back at the old days of Hippocrates, Galen, Percival, Avicenna, al-Ruhawi, al-Razi and others, medicine and ethics were considered inseparable, whereas the modern-day medical profession,[3] it can be argued, is marked by an intellectual schizophrenia which is turning the Hippocratic oath into a *hypocritical oath*. The case described above indicates that some physicians who are role models to students and have taken the solemn oath pledging to protect life and relieve suffering are faltering and abusing a power bestowed upon them by virtue of their profession.

Medicine is inherently a moral enterprise, as a number of authors have argued.[4] It is a profession grounded in the covenant of trust, performed according to a specific set of beliefs about what is right or wrong in medical behavior. Every judgment that a physician makes entails both fact-based and value-based judgments. Medicine is

---

3. Generally speaking, a profession consists of a group of people who hold on to some form of high moral benchmark. They are accepted by the public as possessing a special kind of knowledge and a special set of skills. The profession consists of an organized, educated, and trained collection of people who are ready to exercise their knowledge and skills in the interest of others. A person who belongs to the profession of medicine is someone who, essentially, has been trained in the healing arts and has received a license to practice. Nowadays, one can argue that, in addition to that, he should also be fully dedicated to the ethical principles and values of the medical profession and serve the internal ends of medicine, which are presented in this book. These characteristics, it is maintained, are universal and not context dependant. More will be said about this in the discussion of universalism and social constructionism.

4. Jotterand (2003), Sulmasy (2006), and Pellegrino (2006), among others.

directed towards a healing relationship that requires moral accountability. Hence, a physician is morally and scientifically obligated to act in the best interests of the sick person; failing to do that by acting out of self-interest or commercial gain is failing to live up to the expectations and standards of the profession of medicine. Morality arises with one's interactions with the "other." Physicians constantly interact with patients, their families, other members of healthcare teams, various social entities such as insurance companies, and officials of different organizations. In fact, the therapeutic relationship that marks the physician-patient relationship necessitates some sort of moral accountability that we do not see with the hairdresser, the shoemaker, or the pilot. As such, while considering what she ought to do in a particular situation, the physician must think in terms of values, virtues, morals, and social dynamics. Although scientific considerations are important, they are not the only considerations that matter. The hairdresser interacts with people,[5] yet one does not normally consider hairdressing to be a moral enterprise.[6] There is a difference between the person who enters the hairdresser's shop asking for a hairstyle, for example, and one who enters a clinic or an emergency department of a hospital seeking medical help. The physician affects the patient in a way that the hairdresser or the shoemaker does not, as the physician's activities are entrenched in moral concerns. The duties of the hairdresser are to make sure that she cuts the hair of her client appropriately and perhaps creatively, as well as possibly to ensure that she uses a non-toxic shampoo, but she need not be concerned with why the client wants a new hairstyle. On the other hand, the physician is bound by moral constraints: she has moral liberty to do only that which she has reason to believe will benefit her patient, in the special sense of the term, as an act that results in an "essential good" that promotes well-being. Failure to do so means that she has violated her part of the contract and may be blamed for it. Such is not the case with the hairdresser. The blame facing the physician is a moral one, directed at her skill, ethics, and sense of justice. The blame facing the hairdresser who gives a bad haircut is not a moral blame, although it might be social, aesthetic, or even simply an attack on that hairdresser's expertise. Although one can argue that just as patients trust physicians with their health, clients trust the hairdresser with their hair, what really differentiates the two is that the physician is bound by the duty of beneficence, in the moral sense, while the hairdresser is not. At most, the hairdresser has to fulfill the

---

5. Hairdressing is a business; the end, or purpose, of the hairdresser is to dress the hair of his client. He does not have the well-being of the other in mind as an end in itself.

6. One might argue that nursing and education are such enterprises. Education is particularly interesting as it is concerned with the selves of students in particular and with society at large. Teaching involves a moral action and educators are, or ought to be, moral agents.

demands of her work. In contrast, physicians see patients, perform investigations, diagnose, prescribe, treat, conduct research, and teach. Each and every one of these steps has an important ethical component.

A question that arises concerns which features of the profession of medicine are an essential part of its nature, which are not, and how we distinguish between the two. Essentialism is generally defined as the belief in essences. Thus, essentialism requires that given entities have certain fixed properties that define them and make them what they are. These properties are not accidental characteristics; rather, they are necessary in that the object possessing them cannot exist without them. For example, the property of being human is an essential property that Socrates possesses. So what is or are the essential property or properties of the profession of medicine without which it ceases to be what it is? In an attempt to answer this question, physicians usually begin by listing a set of behaviors that people in other professions do not engage in. For example "a physician deals with health and body while others do not," "in medicine, the patients will inform you of their most personal issues," and "you do physical exams." If an essential characteristic of an object is something that it "must" have, and without which it ceases to be what it is, then the essential characteristics of medicine are not easy to define.

According to Daniel Sokol, the essential characteristic of medicine is love (2008, 1163). Some may consider Sokol to be a bit too optimistic. However, one can argue that what distinguishes medicine from other professions is that patients trust their physicians with their lives. While one might argue that a passenger trusts a pilot with his life, this is not the essence of the passenger-pilot relationship. Rather, it is more of an accidental property, as the trust that happens to exist in this relationship may well be lacking for another passenger. He might trust one airline more than another because of its reputation, but the reason he takes the trip with that airline is because he wants to reach a particular destination. Entrusting the airline with his life takes second place here. In contrast, trust is primary and essential to both medicine and the physician-patient relationship; trust is at the very heart of the medical profession. However, one can imagine a situation where the medical profession is not trusted: misdiagnosis is one leading cause of trust erosion. Another leading cause of distrust resides in the system itself. A *JAMA* article by Barbara Starfield (2000) reveals how the US healthcare system actually contributes to ill health. There are stories of physicians harvesting organs from homeless patients to sell them to patients without the former's consent or knowledge, and there are reports of physicians favoring some private patients over other non-paying ones. So the argument that "trust" is the essence of medicine can falter. Trust ought to be the essence of medicine, and it may have been the essence in the past, but it can no longer be counted on. The problem with this last contention is that it implies that essences change with time. If that is so, are they still essences or have they become something else? This book is not about essences and their nature, and as such, no in-depth discussion addresses this issue, but it is important to recognize that trust is an essential aspect of the physician-patient relationship, and without it the encounter falters in that it does not live up to the ends of medicine. I contend that this relationship is at the heart of medicine and hence, trust is an essential characteristic of the field. The fact that many things are happening that are tarnishing this essence does not mean that it is not a defining essence, but only means that something wrong is taking place and needs to be remedied. If patients don't trust their physicians, something critical is missing in the medical relationship, and the clinical encounter is wanting. One might even question whether the encounter between the patient and the physician would take place at all. Yet despite medical mistakes, most patients act on the conviction that these happen in spite of the physician, and most are confident that the physician will do her utmost to act with the patient's best interest in mind.

Another essential characteristic of the profession of medicine that is inherent in the physician-patient relationship is empathy, or profound appreciation of another's—in this case, the patient's—situation and point of view. One can even argue that what Sokol referred to as "love" (2008) is actually the deep sense of empathy that good physicians are capable of feeling. The hairdresser, the bodyguard, and the pilot can be skilled and all-loving, but they need not be empathetic. Empathy does not define a good pilot, a good bodyguard, or a good hairdresser. It is, however, a defining characteristic of the good physician because health is about the personal narrative of the patient, not only the disease; it is about the patient who suffers from an illness, taking into account the psycho-spiritual-social dimension of illness and healing. A physician, as opposed to a skilled practitioner, treats the patient, not only the disease. She is in touch with the humanity of the ill person. A non-empathetic physician is reduced to the status of a skilled practitioner.

Other characteristics that might characterize the profession of medicine—such as it being based on a fiduciary relationship, centered on confidentiality, and committed to scientific knowledge—are equally essential. One can go on discussing the vital traits of what constitutes the profession of medicine; however, for the sake of this book, suffice to say that the above-mentioned essential characteristics make medicine a unique profession with a unique oath, and this is precisely why neophyte physicians need to be trained and educated in the appropriate virtues in order to become physicians in the fullest sense of the term, and not only skilled technicians or practitioners. The duties of a physician are dictated by the "internal ends" of the profession,[7] and they ought not to violate the dictates of morality; hence the presence of oaths and codes. Medicine is a moral enterprise founded on the covenant of the physician-patient relationship. It is not a business or a commodity that is subject to the whims of the market, and while occasionally it is perceived as such, it ought not be. Rather, it must be guided by a commitment to what is morally right and essentially good, not just by what is necessary in academic or economic undertakings. As such, it invokes ethical principles and must apply them. Medical acts must be recognized as moral practices, geared towards the benefit of the patient, who is viewed as an end in himself. Values enter into almost every decision that a physician makes, and one can argue that medicine imposes collective responsibilities on all its practitioners. In this view, the quintessential moral attribute stems from a conception of the ends of medicine. We therefore need to ask ourselves: what is the nature of medicine, and what are its ends?

1.3. Edmund Pellegrino and the Ends of Medicine

In what follows, I will begin by presenting some of Pellegrino's major ideas, with an emphasis on the thoughts presented in his "The Internal Morality of Clinical Medicine: A Paradigm Shift for the Ethics of the Helping and Healing Professions" (2001a). I will then raise a few questions regarding some of his views that I find controversial or, more precisely, what I consider to be internal inconsistencies in some of his ideas. I will also attempt to resolve them from Pellegrino's point of view. When this is not possible, I will provide an alternative solution in line with Pellegrino's thinking.

---

7. Generally, a profession refers to an occupation which professes to have a knowledge system in a special area, such as health as the basis of the profession of medicine. According to Robert Young, the concept of profession refers to a category that some occupations reach while others do not. Hence, a profession has certain characteristics, and these have certain consequences for those people with professional status and for the establishments at which they work. Young presents six such implications: they spend most of their time in that occupation; their occupation is a calling; they are set aside by signs, symbols, and rewards; their practice depends on special knowledge or skill; they are expected to possess a service orientation; and they benefit from an autonomy limited only by their professional responsibility (Young 1987, 12). The fact remains that it is not easy to give a definition of the concept of "profession." Yet, as Kenneth Calman points out, "it is likely to have some or all of the following characteristics. It is a vocation or calling and implies service to others; it has a distinctive knowledge base which is kept up to date; it determines its own standards and sets its own examinations; it has a special relationship with those whom it serves—patients, clients; it has particular ethical principles—the ethical base; it is self-regulating; and is accountable to patients and to the profession itself." (Calman 1994, 1140).

In his very thorough account of the history of medicine, Pellegrino wrote: "In the earliest times and still in primitive societies, medicine is identified with religion and magic. In the Greek era, medicine first merged with philosophy as well as religion. Aristotle's treatise *On Ancient Medicine* sharply delineated it as a practical endeavor separate from philosophical speculation. Varro, the Roman encyclopedist, classified medicine with the humanities" (Pellegrino 1979, 189–90). Hence, is medicine an art or a science? To claim that medicine is not a science is ridiculous. After all, medicine deals with clinical problems, uses research methods and experimental studies, works with hypotheses, and is often evidence-based, like other sciences.[8] Yet, while medicine is a science, it is also an art—a set of emotional skills acquired by experience and observation. Indeed, physicians come to interact with what is most sensitive in the lives of patients and embark on different kinds of activities which are not scientific, but spring from empathy, and are essential to the practice of medicine as a science. Not only do physicians look after their patients, but they also communicate with them, listen to them, and reassure them, trying their best to understand and support them. The art of medicine is that which allows a physician to explain to family members why the science of medicine did not yield the results they had hoped for, as when a surgery has failed or has resulted in serious complications. It is the art of medicine that helps the physician deal with a patient who is rendered emotionally frail because of his illness. It is this very same art that allows the physician to break bad news, to educate patients and families about the importance of a procedure to which they initially objected, to help them cope with denial, and to comfort family members who lose a loved one. It is this art that encourages a noncompliant patient to return to the same physician for consultations, knowing that the physician will handle him with care and will deal with him appropriately. To put it simply, the art of medicine is that which allows the physician to take care of both the patient and the disease which, in the profession of medicine, should be seen as inseparable. As Joseph Katz puts it, "A medical man was an artist in his ministrations to the ill" (1951, 398).

Unlike other basic sciences, medicine has an extra dimension that makes it a hybrid discipline: Medicine implies that there is a *physician who is dealing directly with living people*, and this in itself marks one of its major departures from other sciences like biology, physics, or chemistry, as the activities of the "pure" sciences will only have an eventual impact on people.

---

8. Edmund Pellegrino and David Thomasma speak of medicine as a "science of practice, a set of principles governing the art of healing" (1981, 7) which combines knowledge with skill in healing.

This brings us to a second feature of medicine. Pellegrino asserts that the notion of humanism encompasses a cognitive as well as an affective element: the cognitive is related to the physician as a human being, a member of society, and a possessor of ideas and modes of expression; while the latter, the affective element, relates to the physician and her feelings and attitudes toward her patients qua persons undergoing the "existential trials of illness" (1979, 157).

This second characteristic of the physician cannot be overestimated. Several studies have revealed humanism as an important, albeit lacking, character trait in modern-day physicians (Arawi 2010; Bazrafkan et al. 2008; Carroll et al. 1998; Wensing and Jung 1998). This view of medicine as belonging to both the sciences and the arts has a bearing on education and what has come to be known as the "philosophy of medicine".[9] Thus, Pellegrino wrote one of his most famous statements defining medicine as "the most humane of the sciences, the most empiric of arts, and the most scientific of humanities" (1979, 17). Notwithstanding, back in 1969, he had posed the presentiment:

> *Medicine, posited between the sciences and the humanities, is one of man's most potent instruments of enlarging both his individual and his social being. To serve this purpose, medicine must respond to the current challenges by creating a new unity of its scientific, ethical and social perspectives. If it does, it might become the genius of that new humanism the world so desperately needs to make technology ever the servant of human purpose (1969, 55).*

It follows from this conception of the nature and function of medicine that the profession of medicine and its practitioners exist to help patients, that medicine is a goal-directed activity conducted by the healthcare practitioner who has a therapeutic role to play. This activity is mainly related to patient care, and in this sense, the welfare and interest of the patient are the outcome the healthcare practitioner is supposed to bring about. Thus, while the sculptor's goal is the production of a statue for its creative worth, the goal of a physician is delineated by the interest of the patient. Medicine is a goal-directed activity that aims towards something external to it and outside the confines of the personal interests of the physician herself. If

---

9. As defined by Pellegrino, the philosophy of medicine "consists in a critical reflection on the matter of medicine—on the content, method, concepts and presuppositions peculiar to medicine *as medicine*." (1998, 325)

the ends—in other words, goals—of this activity are not achieved, the activity itself becomes meaningless.[10]

When talking about the ends of medicine, certain terms cannot be ignored. These include medicine, health, sickness, patients, and doctors. Medicine (from the Latin *medicus*: a helper who carries out the art of curing) is generally thought of when there is a person who is sick and needs his health restored. In order to achieve this goal, he resorts to visiting a physician. Health allows a person to pursue, *ceteris paribus*, his rational plan of life. A patient (from the Latin *patior*—"to suffer"[11]—in the sense of suffering pain and being capable of enduring) is a person who is vulnerable, whose autonomy has somehow been reduced and who is in need of a physician.[12] The physician is in a position of power[13] since she has the knowledge and the skill to heal, and is sought for help by the weak and the vulnerable. The profession of medicine is based on the clinical encounter between patient and physician, hence the importance of the physician-patient relationship. Consequently, Pellegrino notes in most of his writings and lectures that the main ends of medicine have to do with the activity that aims at healing the patient and restoring his health when this is possible.[14] When it is not, this activity has to be directed to relieving the
patient's pain.

Pellegrino also argues that morality is integral to the practice of medicine. In his "The Internal Morality of Clinical Medicine," he traces the concept of an internal morality of the professions back to Fuller, who used it in his philosophy of law, and

---

10. Indeed, there exist what I would like to call the "wrong", or misplaced, goals of medicine—goals that are becoming widespread. For example, if one asks students of medicine why they wish to join the profession, they often give answers focused on gaining prestige or making money. These are examples of "wrong ends." Ends like these distort the profession of medicine and render it more like a business. They undermine the very nature of the profession.

11. Pellegrino rightly argues that suffering cannot be understood solely from the physician's perspective. This is an important aspect of his philosophy, for if a physician were to assume that she knows the suffering of a patient, she still would not be able to understand the personal experience of the patient, just as it is often wrong to assume that the physician can know the quality of life from that patient's perspective. We often tell our medical students how important it is to put themselves at the other end of the stethoscope, knowing that this is not an easy thing to do. Often the person's view of suffering involves his existential being and personal values. Patients must be asked what suffering consists of for them. The results might be surprising for the healthcare practitioner as suffering can have a social, psychological, and spiritual dimension, not only a physiological one. Indeed, an entire new trend in medical ethics has emerged—*narrative medicine*—which takes account of the lived experience of the patient precisely because the particulars of the patient's life are often unknown to the physician and are relevant to the experience of illness. Thus, the notion of suffering, and that it is personal, cannot be separated from the ends of medicine.

12. Interestingly, in Arabic two words are used to denote the term physician: *hakim* (wise) and *tabib* (doctor). The first is mostly used both in spoken and written Arabic and denotes the character of the traditional physician that adds to the duties of the doctor certain moral obligations in addition to her technical expertise and skill.

13. There are several instances where this power can and has been abused. An interesting discussion of the relationship of power to medical ethics can be found in Howard Brody's *The Healer's Power* (New Haven: Yale University Press, 1992).

14. Some might argue that medicine's aim is solely the restoration of the autonomy of the patient. It is my contention that this is a controversial claim for a number of reasons, the most important being that there are a considerable number of patients who suffer an irreversible loss of autonomy in the course of their illnesses—Alzheimer's patients, patients with PVS, and pediatric patients, to name a few. Does this mean that medicine's aim will not be fulfilled with this sample of patients?

argues that it was later modified by John Ladd, who intended an internal morality of medicine to mean a "body of norms binding on physicians by virtue of membership in the profession of medicine" (Pellegrino 2001a, 561). However, Pellegrino does say that his own conception is closer to that of Leon Kass, which was teleologically constructed (2001a, 562). Pellegrino differentiates between what he calls ends that are "external" to medicine and those "internal" to it—for example, healing a sick patient is an end that is internal to medicine whilst receiving payment is an external end (2001a, 559–79). Put simply, the ends of medicine are internal to the profession and can be derived from a correct understanding of the ends of medicine as a practice.[15] He argues that the right norms of the medical practice are *internal* to the profession and henceforth can be derived from the correct discernment of the ends of medicine. External goods are connected to the practice of medicine contingently. Examples of these would be power, wealth, and prestige. These external goods are associated with medicine by chance, not intrinsically, and can be achieved through other means. Any external end that is not compatible with the internal ends of medicine is an intruder to the profession and cannot be accepted as standard practice of the good physician. In other words, and in an Aristotelian approach that ties the *good* to the *end*, once we clearly identify the ends of medicine, we can easily deduce the characteristics of a good physician. Just as a good pianist is one who plays the piano well, a good physician is one who performs her function well by effectively exhibiting the (internal) ends of medicine. Thus, Pellegrino distinguishes between the use of the words *end* (*telos*)—referring to concepts that are internal to medicine, like curing, caring, and healing—and *goal* (or purpose)—referring to concepts that are external, such as torturing prisoners, participating in executions, and performing abortions.[16] This is not to say that goals are, by definition, morally undesirable. For example, abortion can serve the internal ends of medicine when it is done to save the life of the mother. One can even argue that taking part in executions aims to reduce suffering, which can be viewed as one of the aims of medicine. As Pellegrino

---

15. Pellegrino puts a lot of emphasis on the word "profession" as a public declaration and hence a promise to perform the duties of a physician.

16. One might wonder whether there is such a thing as a "bad physician" to begin with, or whether the title physician should be rescinded when a healthcare practitioner performs in a way that is not in line with the internal ends of medicine. The term "good physician" should be considered redundant just as the term "bad physician" is an oxymoron. The point is that a physician is someone who, by definition, should have the best interest of her patient in mind, serve the internal ends of medicine, honor her profession, and be selfless when it comes to her profession. A physician should be virtuous wholeheartedly because one cannot be virtuous only in part. Students of medicine strive to achieve an MD degree that qualifies them to become skilled technicians unless they have that extra "something" that makes them a physician. The fact that an MD does not automatically result in one's being a physician is why there is a need to re-evaluate the medical educational system and to include virtues as an essential part of the education of the neophyte physician. That extra "something" is what makes the medical student aim at serving the internal ends of medicine. There are particular core virtues without which a physician is nothing but a "skilled technician," or what people call a "bad doctor"; they will be addressed shortly. There is no such thing as "bad doctor," Since a doctor, or preferably, a physician, is either good or not. He cannot be bad. It is an oxymoron, a contradiction—like being a thing and its opposite at the same time.

mentions, there are times when goals coincide with the internal ends of medicine yet remain external to the practice. Thus, to be a healthcare practitioner, such as a physician, one has to acknowledge the internal ends of medicine, which are traditionally to cure, care, and help (1999, 57), and Pellegrino emphasizes that it is "healing which is specific to this patient, not healing as an end" (1999, 63). Hence, one can conclude that for Pellegrino, as for others, medicine entails much more than simply "diagnose and treat." It is defined as "knowledge-based and directed by an architectonic principle—healing or helping a sick person become whole again" (1999, 63). As stated in Pellegrino and Thomasma, "the ends of medicine are ultimately the restoration or improvement of health and, more proximately, to heal, that is, to cure illness and disease or, when this is not possible, to care for and help the patient to live with residual pain, discomfort, or disability" (1993, 52–53).

This idea is echoed by Jeremy Sugarman and Daniel Sulmasy (2001, 78–79): "Medicine exists because humans become ill and want to heal, ameliorate, cure, or prevent this universal human frailty." They add that the physician has to serve not only the patient's good, but also the patient's "perception of good—material, emotional or spiritual." (2010, 99). A few years later, Pellegrino adds:

> *[T]he optimal end of healing is the good of the whole person—physical, emotional, and spiritual. The physician, manifestly, is no expert in every dimension. He or she, however, should be alert to the patient's needs in each sphere, do what is within his or her capabilities, and work with others in the healthcare team to come as close as clinical reality permits to meeting the several levels contained in the idea of the good of the patient (2001a, 569).*

At another point, he notes, "The end of healing is the good of the whole person" (2005b, 25). Miller and Brody (2001, 586–99) discuss further the internal morality of medicine, which they define in terms of the "goals of clinical medicine" and argue that there should be a set of duties which constrains medical practice in the pursuit of these goals. We will return to this subject later.

Interestingly, in another article in which he talks about the duties of the physician, Pellegrino notes that "some things ought never to be done" in the profession of medicine (2005a, 469). He argues that certain moral absolutes are inherent in the physician-patient relationship and are necessary for the attainment of the good of the patient, which is ultimately the *telos* of the relationship. Pellegrino refers to

Aristotle's contention that "certain acts were always wrong and should never be done—e.g., murder, adultery, lying, stealing" (2005a, 472). For him, "Clinical moral absolutes are norms and mandates that must never be abrogated because their abrogation vitiates the healing ends of medicine" (2005a, 475). These absolutes which Pellegrino believes are essential to medicine's end are: to act for the good of the patient, not to kill, to keep one's promises, to protect the dignity of the patient, not to lie, and to avoid complicity with evil. However interesting, this idea is quite a controversial one. In what follows, I will raise questions regarding some of Pellegrino's views, as presented above, and I try to respond to them from the point of view of Pellegrino himself. When this is not possible, I strive to provide an alternative theory which is in line with the general framework of Pellegrino's thought.

1.3.1. The Ends of Clinical Medicine

Pellegrino argues that the ends of medicine have to do with healing the patient and restoring his health whenever possible, and that the ends of medicine should aim for the good of the patient without ignoring the patient's own perceptions of his own good. According to Robert Veatch, Pellegrino's belief that the ends of medicine are non-controversial is a false view for the very simple reason that the goals of medicine have changed over time (Veach 2001, 630). Veatch argues that while in the middle of the twentieth century physicians were committed to the preservation of life, with time this evolved into prioritizing a commitment to prolong life, followed by the goals of curing disease and relieving suffering, and more recently, the prevention of disease and the promotion of health. He maintains that these goals have competing claims, with the result that we often find ourselves in controversial situations (2001, 631). However, all four goals highlighted by Veatch have the good of the patient as the ultimate end and the promotion of health as the sole aim, and as such do not contradict Pellegrino's view of the ends of medicine.

Veatch, who argues for an "external morality" of medicine, recounts the dilemma of Internalsville (2001, 632) to show that the ends of medicine are closely tied to the ends of living and social functioning. He asks, "Assuming that Pellegrino has it right when he says that the end of medicine is to promote the health or healing of the patient, does castration serve this objective in Internalsville or does it thwart it?" (2001, 633). Veatch goes on to show that it thwarts it. His argument is that deciding which view of medicine to follow requires a reflection upon basic religious, philosophical, and cultural norms (2001, 632). Yet, one can contend that the role of the physician and the practice of medicine itself have limits that are set by the internal nature of medicine. Although one can argue that a physician who agrees to reduce the size of a woman's breasts to allow her to improve her golf swing or her social status is serving the ends of medicine, one can also contend that the ends served are not the "internal ends" of the profession since ideally the physician violates the body only to heal it. When the opposite happens, one will have to start looking for another definition of medicine and its ends. Although the patient's perceptions are important, the physician cannot be forced to act against her own professional conscience precisely because, to Pellegrino, the key relevant value is beneficence.[17] It becomes questionable to assert that it is morally required that a physician who practices in the Kingdom of Saudi Arabia change her behavior when practicing in the UK or China on the pretext that medicine's morality is externally derived and tied to social function. Would we not be creating morally schizophrenic physicians if we did so? It remains a fact that to many, particularly in the US, autonomy is the most valued principle in contemporary medicine. As such, if the patient wishes to have her breasts reduced, even when aware of all the risks involved, then the physician, although required to warn the patient, has two options. She can either respect the choice of the patient and go ahead with the operation or refer her to another physician who is willing to do it.

In general, putting too much weight on a patient's autonomy may be problematic in many respects. For one, a physician may end up taking the easy way out by simply complying with the decision of the patient—in other words, giving up on the patient under the pretext of his autonomy. The patient's good and the patient's perception of his own good may be different. According to Pellegrino, "what is medically "good" simply on grounds of physiological effectiveness may not be "good" if it violates higher levels of good, like the patient's good as he perceives that good. This perceived good is the second level of patient good" (2001a, 569). He later on defines this good as respecting the patient's "personal preferences, choices and values, and the kind of life he wants to live, the balance he strikes between the benefit and burdens of the proposed intervention," acknowledging that they are "unique for every patient and cannot be defined by the physician, the family or anyone else" (2001a, 569). For Pellegrino, the patient's perceptions of the good supersede the patient's medical good, for "to serve the good as perceived by the patient, the medical good must be

---

17. What counts as beneficence is, for Pellegrino, that which is oriented towards healing and acting for the good of the patient.

placed within the context of this patient's life-plans and life situations" (2001a, 569). This, however, is controversial: If the medical good has to account for the patient's perception of his own good, then the physician will find herself having to respect the wishes of her patient even if those wishes go against the actual medical good of the patient and the beliefs and medical judgment of the physician. So, where do we draw the line? Pellegrino finds a way out of this conundrum by arguing that the patient's good is superseded by the "good for humans" and that the physician has a concept of the good that may differ from that of the patient. In this case, the physician is not forced to cooperate with the patient and can simply say that she is not the right doctor for him: "[w]hen the patient's and physician's values are sharply at variance, the physician should decline to enter the relationship or withdraw from it graciously, with candor, and without recrimination" (Pellegrino and Thomasma 1993, 76).

The bottom line is that the inherent and absolute dignity of the patient forbids the physician from imposing her concept of the good on the patient at any of the four levels, except in the case of medical good in an emergency. Indeed, Pellegrino is aware of the problematic issues raised by emphasizing the importance of a patient's perceptions of the good. He elaborates that the physician is not obliged to do whatever the patient defines as good because this would make the "patient's perception of the good "dominant over all other goods. It would make patient preference morally and lexically superior to the medical good, the good for humans, and the spiritual good" (2001a, 571), which, in my opinion and that of Pellegrino, is not what ought to be the case. It remains true that it is not clear how deliberations happen and how the conflict between the levels of the good is solved. Yet, one solution would be to rely on the practical wisdom of the physician, to resort to the "rational good" explained below, or to have a form of *prima facie* good *following* W. D. Ross.[18]

One should also note that, for many physicians, the ends of medicine are different. They vary from prevention and healing of illness to improving health, prolonging life, giving hope, and serving the best interest of the patient. The "Hastings Report on the Goals of Medicine" refers to five major goals: promoting health, reducing certain kinds of pain and suffering, fighting disease and injury, advancing the quality of life, and saving and prolonging life (Callahan 1996). In line with that report, Pellegrino was aware that redefining the ends of medicine would become the central problem in the philosophy of medicine and he questioned whether physicians should be

---

18. W. D. Ross (1877–1971), a Scottish philosopher known for his work in ethics.

"healers or servants of societal good, businesspeople, entrepreneurs, bureaucrats, scientists" (2005b, 21), or something else. For him, as previously noted, the main ends of medicine have to do with what aims at healing the patient and restoring his health whenever this is possible. There might be other peripheral ends that can be functions of culture and/or time, but the core ends are, and indeed ought to be, unchangeable. For those who contend that the ends of medicine ought to be the restoration of autonomy, one can argue that Pellegrino's view also incorporates that, of course, assuming that it is a patient whose autonomy we are able to restore. Restoring the health of the patient is restoring his autonomy, which was initially fractured by the fact of illness. Add to this that the second level of the good, detailed a little further below, honors autonomy, and Pellegrino argues that this level of the good supersedes the patient's perception of the good.

Nevertheless, there remains the issue of patients who have autonomous requests for abortion or euthanasia. Pellegrino is a conservative on both abortion and euthanasia, believing that autonomy can be rightly limited when it is a question of taking a life. Pellegrino would not honor such requests because they do not respect the "spiritual good" and, furthermore, doctors must not kill. Arguing from a Roman Catholic standpoint, he views euthanasia as murder and wrong regardless of whether the intention is to relieve suffering or anything else, regardless of the circumstances. According to the late Pope John Paul II, "euthanasia is an attack on life that no human authority can justify, because the life of an innocent person is an indispensable good" (1998). The same idea was reaffirmed by Pope Benedict, who stressed "the firm and constant ethical condemnation of all forms of direct euthanasia, in keeping with the centuries-long teaching of the Church" (Catholic News Agency 2008). From their perspective, euthanasia violates the love and justice humans owe to God and man. Life is a gift from God, and no one has a right to intentionally take it away. This is an argument that might very well be accepted by most Christians as well as Muslims and members of other faiths. One can argue that there is some discrepancy in Pellegrino's argument because respecting the will of the patient and his autonomy logically and necessarily entails respecting his advance directive, living will, or wish for euthanasia and abortion. Persons have a fundamental human right to make personal choices about matters related to life and death. Euthanasia and abortion are thought of as part of a continuum of means of exercising one's freedom of choice and "right to die." In 1991, a 45-year-old leukemic patient named Diane asked Dr. Timothy Quill to give her a barbiturates prescription which would enable her to put an end to her pain and misery at a time of her choosing (Quill 1991). To many, by doing so Quill was acting in Diane's best interests and respecting her rights. At his trial, he was actually acquitted although physician-assisted suicide was forbidden in the State of New York. An autonomous being has the right to choose, and this right has to be respected, even to the point of indifference as to whether this choice is religiously right or wrong. Pellegrino cannot have it both ways. He would argue that such a patient would have to find another physician, but this is morally worrisome, for it is a form of abandoning the patient when the patient needs the physician the most, and it betrays a long-established physician-patient relationship. This leads us back to the question raised above: Are medicine's ends universal or are they socially constructed?

1.4. Towards a Combined View of the Ends of Medicine

One of the important issues that arises regarding the ends of medicine is whether these ends are universal, applying to all human beings, or socially constructed. In what follows, I argue that the ends of medicine are neither solely universal, as Pellegrino argues, nor are they simply socially constructed. Rather, it is my contention that the ends of medicine are universal in the sense that they operate within a universal framework, but that they also are socially constructed in that they are liable to change and evolve depending on the society and the times. Having said that, it is important to note that these core values may occasionally conflict, and when this happens, the physician will have to use her practical wisdom to decide what her actual duties are in each specific case. One is tempted to maintain that if they are universal, then there are certain core traits and values that students of medicine should be taught so that they can rightly serve the ends of medicine. While, if these ends are socially constructed, then the question of such core traits, although they might still hold, may become less stringent and be replaced by something more culturally relative; I beg to differ. Although a universalist view of the ends of medicine would emphasize the importance of teaching core values and traits to students of medicine, the same applies even if one believes that the ends of medicine are socially constructed. Because medicine is a moral endeavor, founded on a covenant of trust and operating within a framework of right and wrong, as elaborated earlier,[19] one can say that, *ceteris paribus*, some things cannot be done in the practice of medicine without violating the internal ends of the profession.

---

19. See chapter 1, section 1.2.

Given the nature of the profession, medicine's internal ends lie in the good of the person seeking help, and this is, universally, healing and helping, regardless of time and place.[20] The ends of medicine embody a reaction to a universal human experience, which is illness. The fact that medicine has internal ends further highlights this universal dimension: these ends transcend the limits of the *here* and *now* precisely because they are a function of the clinical encounter and the existential nature of illness and its consequences. They defy space and time because sickness is a universal plight and the patient entrusts the physician with his health. But I would argue that these internal ends function as moral boundaries that also provide a universal framework in that they apply to all physicians everywhere and at all times. Social constructions exist and operate within that framework. The particular circumstances and individual differences and contexts of an illness may vary, yet the nature of the experience itself is the common denominator. This experience and the existential crisis it creates are reflected in numerous codes of medical ethics across geography and history. The codes from all the cultures and periods of time, including our own, reflect different societies and norms but have common guidelines which identify the healing of the sick as being the primary goal of the medical profession. These common guidelines reflect the moral boundaries and the universal nature of these ends. They are the framework within which the social constructions operate. Needless to say, codes are born situationally and contextually; they do not come into being *ex-nihilo*. Medicine has its purpose, and physicians have their integrity. This purpose and this integrity cannot and indeed should not be derived from something external to the profession of medicine. If this were to happen, it would be the end of the profession of medicine as we know it: medicine would become the slave of external social forces that could very easily damage its reputation and its raison d'être. Yet, one cannot ignore the fact that societal values and culture affect the physician and the profession. To begin with, everyday relationships among human beings are socially constructed, and what is accepted in one society often is not in another. I am not advocating cultural relativism; rather I am simply stating a historical fact. The same applies to the physician-patient encounter. Certain societies dictate that only a female physician can examine a female patient except in cases of dire emergencies and a lack of female physicians. In some cultures, it is acceptable, indeed required, that physicians be honest and upfront with their patients when it comes to diagnosis and prognosis, while in others, this is seen as utter insensitivity

---

20. Physicians might have additional secondary or external ends in their pursuit of medicine, yet none of these ends define medicine's primary or internal end.

and a lack of moral decorum.[21] In certain cultures, pregnancies of unmarried women are terminated; in others, the unmarried expectant mother is killed, as her pregnancy is considered a breach of honor.[22] Certain rural areas refuse to believe that an X-ray or MRI is adequate evidence, and insist on a physical exam. Some rely on insurance and state money for treatment; others rely on family and friends. Indeed, one can even argue that what is counted as a malady may vary over time and can be subject to differing interpretations. Kevin Wildes argues that one cannot ignore the social dimension of medicine (Wildes 2001). He asserts that medicine is socially constructed; in other words, medicine is practiced in a certain social or cultural context which cannot be ignored. Pellegrino agrees that medicine is practiced in social or cultural contexts yet denies "that this entails social construction as the method for defining the ends or goals of medicine" (Pellegrino 2001b, 177).

For Pellegrino, contending that medicine is practiced within a social context, as Wildes does, implies that one can derive the meaning of medicine from the social context. Yet, this is not the case, Wildes argues, because "[m]edicine comes into existence in the clinical encounters or in public health when knowledge of the sciences basic to medicine is employed for a specific end—i.e., for the cure or containment of illness in humans and society" (Wildes 2001, 77). The main problem with Pellegrino's restrictive universalist view is the fact that he distinguishes medicine from other professions by the fact that it is centered on the encounter of the physician with each individual patient, and he derives the essence of medicine from this one-to-one encounter. The fact is that a contemporary clinical encounter is far from being a one-to-one encounter. Other physicians and members of the healthcare team often are present, as are the insurance company—albeit in a different form—and the state, legislators, hospital administration, and others. Social structures make this encounter achievable. Even disease is socially constructed in the sense that social meaning is attached to the underlying biological condition. For example, in certain cultures, STDs, AIDS, mental illnesses, and syphilis are stigmatized, and even this stigma can change over time.[23] This has repercussions on the pronouncing of illness and access to treatment, as well as on social ramifications. This is an example of how medicine is affected by the values of the culture in which it is being practiced. Pellegrino sees medicine as extending beyond culture, which, to the reader, can be seen as a "metaphysication of medicine," if one may be allowed the expression. To Pellegrino, social construction allows for some distorted forms of medicine and

---

21. These differences existed in ancient times as well.
22. This is why in certain cultures physicians often debate the morality of hymenoplasty.
23. See Conrad and Barker, "The Social Construction of Illness," S67–S79.

medical ethics like those developed under German National Socialism, Stalinist Russia, and other authoritarian regimes. A socially constructed philosophy of medicine would be alien to the ends of medicine. Yet, one can argue that what was done under those regimes was wrong and that what the physicians of those regimes did amounted to a failure to honor the moral boundaries of medicine. Thus, the burden of proof falls upon those who have failed to do what is right.

Now, why accept Pellegrino's essentialist view of the ends of medicine, and not Miller's and Brody's evolutionary view? They argue that Pellegrino's conception is an "essentialist"[24] one in that he reduces the goals and ends of medicine to platonic forms that are "historically unchanging" (Miller and Brody 2001, 584). They disagree with Pellegrino because they distrust the platonic forms and consider his conception to be essentially a conservative one. As such, they present what they call an "evolutionary conception of the internal morality of medicine", which is an outcome of a dialectic between essentialism and social constructivism (2001, 585). They do not derive the internal morality of medicine from a constant conception of the practice of medicine which yields a single set of goals and ends that applies at all times and in all places. Rather, for them, the nature of medicine and its internal norms are evolving, and this evolution occurs in dialogue with the adjoining culture such that the goals of medicine develop alongside human history and culture. Consequently, medicine may from time to time be reconceptualized, and can thus assimilate new behaviors and duties on the part of physicians. Contemplating the traditional goals of medicine leads Miller and Brody to conclude that there is a "historical continuity," or evolution, to the goals of medicine. This evolution can, for example, include the participation of some physicians in helping some of their terminally ill patients to end their lives through physician-assisted suicide, or euthanasia. It is my contention that while this evolutionary view might appeal to a moral pluralist, it does not really hold without affecting the nature of the profession of medicine in its quintessence. So, in a way, one can argue for a fusion of the essentialist and the evolutionary theories.

In what follows, an amendment to the evolutionary view is proposed that takes account of Pellegrino's essentialist conception. Although one cannot deny the fact that the goals of medicine and the duties of physicians are affected by the culture and the times, one can maintain that the evolutionary conception does not necessarily

---

24. Miller and Brody argue that Pellegrino sees this as the only possible substitute for a *socialist constructionist* conception of medicine according to which "medicine and its morality can be reinvented more or less at whim whenever external social forces pushed it in new directions" (2001, 585).

do away with the essentialist position presented by Pellegrino. New goals and new duties do arise as a result of context and developments;[25] after all, physicians in ancient times did not have to worry about issues resulting from IVF, stem cell research, or cloning precisely because such technologies were non-existent. The contention being made here is that there are *core* duties and *core* goals that remain static, unchanged regardless of time and culture, and that these core duties and goals are part of the internal morality of medicine and define the profession of medicine.[26] There is an unchanging crucial core of medical morality surrounded by a periphery that is subject to change through interaction and dialogue with the neighboring culture, society, and times, and such peripheral goals may serve purposes other than healing.[27] Some examples include elective cosmetic surgery, participation in interrogation, and fertility enhancement. Which dynamic goals to assign to the periphery is not an easy thing to decide and will have to be a product of deliberation by concerned thinkers and ethicists. It is essential, though, that throughout these deliberations, core values—such as the healing of the patient and the integrity of the physician—should not be compromised. The relative weight of each is another issue altogether. Therefore, Pellegrino did have a point in arguing that medicine has certain goals and duties that are internal to it, and these core goals and duties are not a function of culture and time. The problem with his theory lies in the fact that he left it at that and failed to see that medicine cannot remain blind to social and cultural developments, particularly since the needs of patients are often a function of such developments. On the practical level, this taking account of social changes and developments is seen in the amendments and developments of new codes of medical ethics and new versions of the Hippocratic oath. One cannot turn a blind eye to the fact that the social fabric is powerful, and medicine is about people and society. Inevitably, medicine is a function of people and society.

The amendment I am offering is not immune to criticism. One can argue that there is no essential core that is impervious to socially constructed changes, be it in terms of goals or duties, and that whatever has remained from history has been retained as a matter of contingency yet may still change with time and cultural or social interaction. A response to this would be that some factor inherent in the nature of the profession itself and closely tied to its goals "requires" that the core duties or

---

25. One wonders whether there are any goals and duties that get dropped. The ends of medicine have always been the same. Only with the advancement of modern technology are new goals added. Practically, some duties have been dropped. For example, physicians often omit physical examinations and send their patients directly to an X-Ray machine, but whether this should be the case is another matter altogether.

26. "Core" signifying basic, essential, and unchanging.

27. Peripheral goals being a function of time and place. They vary depending on context, culture, evolution, technological development, and other factors.

goals remain unchanged. Core goals and core duties necessarily remain unchanged, otherwise medicine would become something else. This factor constitutes its *essence*, so to speak. Other *evolutionary ends* are bound to arise with time precisely because medical technology is developing at a rapid pace and new issues are emerging in the clinical encounter. However, *core ends*, like beneficence, are such that they can only be trumped by reasons that serve the ends of medicine. The alternative is that medicine ceases to be a healing profession. These core ends are the focal point around which everything else in the medical profession revolves, and they represent a stable foundation that allows trust in the physician to thrive and develop. Yet situations may arise when, in order to benefit the patient, physicians find themselves sliding towards what can arguably be viewed as harmful to the patient, such as morphine used to relieve suffering at the end of a patient's life, which can also hasten death by suppressing his respiratory system. In such cases, the principle of double effect helps one make decisions.[28] However, the appeal to *phronesis*, or practical wisdom, is required to resolve any conflict that might arise between different core ends.

1.5. Needs, Perceptions, and the Ends of Medicine

According to Pellegrino, "the optimal end of healing is the good of the whole person, encompassing the physical, emotional, and spiritual. The physician, manifestly, is no expert in every dimension. He or she, however, should be alert to the patient's *needs* in each sphere,[29] do what is within his or her capabilities, and work with others on the healthcare team to come as close as clinical reality permits to meeting the several levels contained within the idea of the good of the patient" (2001a, 569). It is here that Pellegrino introduced the notion of "needs." Needs and perceptions are two different things. In a moral sense, one can argue that the object of *need* can be viewed objectively as a thing that a person possesses—e.g., I need food in order to survive. In the absence of the object of need, harm will ensue—e.g., if I do not eat over a period of time, I will die.[30] Perceptions, on the other hand, can be viewed as subjective. A person might perceive his good to be X when in reality it is Y. A patient might perceive that it is better for him not to take iron pills because they are causing him stomach cramps when, in fact, he is severely anemic and will face a serious physiological loss

---

28. The doctrine of double effect stipulates that if doing what is deemed morally good has a morally bad consequence or side effect, it is ethically acceptable to do it as long as the side effect was not intended to begin with. A typical example would be if a physician gives a certain medication to a patient in an attempt at alleviating his suffering, knowing that doing this might shorten the life of the patient.

29. My emphasis.

30. Hence, one needs food, but desires cheesecake.

of function should he leave his anemia untreated. The assumption here is that health is a "good" that patients look for; they seek the help of the physician to restore their health. It may be a view of health defined by the values of patients, but there are some general parameters of objectivity that constitute health for all; that severe anemia will damage the body is one of them. Readers of Pellegrino might confuse the word "needs," as used above, as being an objective need as opposed to a subjective perception of the patient. However, Pellegrino is referring to the physical need as the medical good of the patient, the emotional need as the perception of the patient, and the spiritual need as the spiritual good of the patient. Once this is clarified, ambiguity disappears. Pellegrino argues that "the medical good of the patient is a four-tiered idea: the medical good, the patient's perception of the good, the good for humans as the kind of thing humans are, and the spiritual good."[31] Earlier he proposed a theory where different kinds of goods supersede one another. The medical good is important and "aims at the return of physiological function of mind and body, the relief of pain and suffering, by medication, surgical interventions, psychotherapy, etc." (2001a, 569). This good must, however, "be brought into proper relationship with the other levels of the patient's good. Otherwise, it may become harmful" (2001a, 569). It is superseded by the patient's perception of his good, which has to do with the patient's "personal preferences, choices, and values, and the kind of life he wants to live, the balance he strikes between the benefit and burdens of the proposed intervention" (2001a, 569). Both—the medical good and the patient's perceptions of the good—are superseded by the "good for humans as humans." This, he argues, was the good Aristotle wanted to define as the *telos* of human life (2001a, 570). At the level of the good for humans as humans, the familiar principles of medical ethics proposed by James Childress and Tom Beauchamp are taken into account (2001). Pellegrino argues that "in the clinical encounter, the medical good and the personal good must, in their turn, be consistent with and protect the good for human beings as humans" (2001a, 570). The questions that arise here are: What if physicians are not capable of ensuring that? What happens then? What if, say, the medical good of the patient indicates that abortion is in the best interest of the patient, while the patient's perception of her good—her personal good—is that she keeps the baby? How can they protect and be consistent with the human good when, to begin with, they contradict each other? Pellegrino's solution to this problem is to resort to the spiritual good, the paramount good that supersedes all. The "spiritual good" is the highest level of good which must be served in the clinical encounter and this is "the good of the patient as

---

31. Pellegrino, personal communication, 18 October 2010.

a spiritual being—i.e., as one who, in his own way, acknowledges some end to life beyond material well-being" (2001a, 570). At this point we are in the realm of the spirit, however differently this may be defined by different people. If it violates this good, the medical good "could never be a healing act" (2001a, 571). This is a strong claim that renders the medical good dependent on the spiritual good. Moreover, the three examples that Pellegrino states are extreme cases: 1) Blood transfusions in the case of a Jehovah's witness, 2) Abortion of a genetically impaired fetus for a Catholic, and 3) Discontinuance of life support for an Orthodox Jew (2001a, 571). Yet we often encounter controversial cases where physicians face conflicting duties, and the answer is not straightforward. This is all good for those who believe in the existence of the spirit beyond material existence, but what about patients and physicians who do not? Should we stop at the level of the good for humans? In this case, what solves the problem of the conflict between the medical good and the patient's good? Pellegrino's answer is simple. While the physician has to respect the good of the patient, she is a human being, not a "patient-own automaton" and cannot violate her "own moral percept of the good at the pleasure of the patient."[32] Pellegrino continues: "If the patient asks me to violate my conscience, I say politely: 'No. I cannot do what you want. I am not the best doctor for you.'"[33] To some, this might seem to be a morally acceptable alternative. The patient is served, and the physician's professional conscience is not violated. However, I argue that this four-tiered idea, although interesting, puts Pellegrino in a tight spot in that it reveals an inconsistency in his thinking. It seems that each level of the good can lead to more problems than solutions when it comes to dealing with patients. The medical good is the biological good of the patient and, as such, it seems to be the least problematic of them all since it can be decided on a scientific basis. Yet, this good is left subordinate to all the other levels of the good. However, for someone like Pellegrino, who argues that beneficence is a primary end of medicine, this good should, perhaps, supersede all other goods because the medical professional is the one trained to know what is medically better for the patient. The patient's perception of the good can very well be subjective and might conflict with his own medical good. What would or should a conscientious doctor do in that situation? What if the patient's perception of his good is false because this patient has an unscientific belief that will damage his life? Should the physician yield to that conception if, after deliberation and education, the patient still sticks to his false conception of the good? One major difference between medicine and other professions, such as marketing or business, is that in medicine

---

32. Pellegrino, personal communication, 18 October 2010.
33. Ibid.

the patient has minimal sovereignty[34] in asking for what he wishes, and this sovereignty is limited by the knowledge of the physician and the medical condition of the patient. In other words, if a patient comes in asking for nonindicated surgery with high risk and side effects, the conscientious physician should not grant him this request even if the offer is a lucrative one, as is the case with some plastic surgery. Pellegrino says that the patient's conception of the good is superseded by the human good; but who decides what the human good is? Furthermore, even if the boundaries of this human good are universal, some goods remain that are socially constructed, and hence, the physician's view of the human good might come into conflict with the views of the patient and/or other physicians due to their differing backgrounds. What should be done in this case? To simply suggest that the patient resort to another physician becomes a slippery slope. To solve the problem by resorting to the spiritual good which supersedes all goods is even more problematic for at least two reasons: 1) some patients do not believe in any supernatural entity and to them resorting to a spiritual good is useless; 2) it might very well be the case that the supernatural belief system of the physician and that of the patient are incompatible. What should be done in this case? Tell the patient to resort to another physician? Does this mean that, ultimately, patients should be seeing physicians who hold the same cultural and spiritual beliefs as they do in order to ensure better care, at least as they perceive it? This is a dangerous conclusion. Pellegrino, who contends that the heart of the medical encounter is the physician-patient relationship and who gives supremacy to the patient's good, argues that the solution, whenever there is a conflict between a patient and a physician, is to ask the patient to resort to another doctor. This is a form of abandonment of the patient and his good. Perhaps the spiritual good needs to be replaced by the "rational good," this being the good that any rational physician who has internalized the virtues would choose after deliberation. The physician will have to use her *phronesis* and good character to decide what is to be done without morally abandoning the patient and without encumbering herself with actions that conflict with her moral professionalism.

---

34. Sovereignty refers to a person's capacity to determine his own affairs, while autonomy refers to a patient's right to make decisions about his medical care.

1.6. Performing Abortion as an Example of an End External to the Profession of Medicine

As noted previously, Pellegrino contends that beneficence is the primary principle of medical ethics, that healing should be the exclusive goal of medicine, and that acts like abortion and euthanasia are not part of its internal ends. According to him, abortion is an "intrinsically evil act" and, as such, it cannot serve the moral end of healing. It is conceived of as an end external to medicine, one which allows "complicity with evil" (2005a, 481). Yet, one can argue that performing abortions need not be considered as an end external to medicine per se and that Pellegrino pronounced it as such on the basis of his own personal religious beliefs. If abortion is performed in order to save the life of a mother, one can argue that this is very much in line with the internal ends of medicine, that it is done with beneficence in mind, and cannot be said to be done in complicity with evil. The same can be said of an abortion performed on a fetus that suffers severe malformations that are incompatible with life. Such malformations will only cause physical and psychological harm to the child, to her family, and by extension to society.[35] Consider a child with Tay-Sachs, a fatal disease caused by the lack of the hexosaminidase A enzyme. The illness has a genetic origin and, although newborns who suffer from infantile Tay-Sachs look healthy, they will have a life full of suffering and pain; eventually, the illness leads to total paralysis, blindness, and death (Arras 1990, 366). Will preserving the life of this fetus be in line with the ends of medicine, which are to help, heal, and cure?[36] This issue becomes more problematic when prenatal tests intended to detect congenital malformations and chromosomal aberrations—like sonography, first and second trimester blood test screening, amniocentesis, and chorionic villus sampling—are available and are performed on women who can be denied abortions on the grounds that doctors ought not terminate lives. What is the point of having the means to detect abnormalities in utero when a physician is morally bound not to abort? Almost everyone recalls the horrific birth deformities that ensued from the use of the thalidomide drug. Hiroshima's "mushroom cloud" is yet another infamous story that reverberates in the minds of many. In the aftermath of the detonation of atomic bombs in Japan and the ensuing radiation, women gave birth to children with terrible defects. A further example is from Carole Gallagher, quoted by Bryan Taylor, who

---

35. Note that the obstetrician has two patients: the mother and the fetus.

36. There continues to be a lack of universal agreement, and people hold different opinions on what constitutes the minimum requirements for a decent life and what constitutes a malformation that is incompatible with life. It is my contention that before entering into parenthood, parents should ask themselves whether the life that they are begetting will be one that satisfies the fundamentals for decent living, or one of very low quality, surrounded by agony and pain.

relates the following story of a mother and daughter whose lives were badly affected by US government testing of nuclear weaponry:

> *[W]hile she was carrying her daughter in the womb, she was exposed to radioactive fallout that caused nausea, burns, and blisters on her skin and led to the loss of her teeth, hair, fingernails, and toenails. Her daughter was subsequently delivered prematurely, suffering from cancer, and weighing little more than three pounds. At the age of six months, her cancer was treated with crude and unlocalized radiation that deformed her heart, lungs, breasts, and spine. As Diana Lee Woosley aged, she suffered from constant vomiting and congestive heart failure and underwent traumatic surgical procedures to correct her spinal deformity. Her face, we learn, is swollen from large doses of prednisone, which she must take to combat the diseases that exploit her weakened immune system—a treatment that has itself caused diabetes (Taylor 1997, 583).*

If the primary end of medicine is beneficence, serving the good of the patient—the medical end of the physician-patient relationship—the question that automatically follows is: How was the good of Diana Lee Woosely and her mother served when the life that she is leading is pain and agony? Religion and purgation arguments aside, her good has not been served; quite the contrary. Their suffering could have been avoided by an abortion performed at the earliest stages of pregnancy; physical, psychological, and financial torment could have been circumvented.

One can contend that controversial issues like abortion and euthanasia can fall either within the internal or the external realms of ends, depending on the situation, particularly since, as Pellegrino himself states, the end of clinical medicine is caring and curing.[37] Add to this that such actions might serve the good of the patient *as the patient perceives it*, which Pellegrino argues supersedes the medical good. Thus, while the physician can be a conscientious objector, one cannot dismiss abortion altogether as being evil or not part of the internal ends of medicine as Pellegrino perceives them to be. Put simply, if an abortion is performed for the purpose of healing and the good of the patient, it serves the internal ends of medicine. One might argue that abortion might become part of the internal ends of medicine depending on the situation, the medical good, the patient's perception of the good, and the good for humans as humans. The spiritual good is itself grounds for

---

37. See Pellegrino's cogent account against euthanasia in "Doctors must not kill" (1992).

controversy. In certain religions, abortions are permissible at certain times and in certain conditions. For example, Islam allows abortions if the fetus is deformed, provided that abortion takes place prior to ensoulment, which is usually said to be at 120 days of pregnancy. After that, abortion is allowed only if the pregnancy causes danger to the life of the mother. In 2008, al-Azhar—considered to be the highest Muslim Sunni seat of learning—declared a fatwa to the effect that a woman made pregnant by rape can abort as soon as she knows that she is pregnant. For the Roman Catholic Church, the fetus is a person at the moment of conception, and abortion is a mortal sin. Judaism does not forbid abortion altogether, particularly during the first forty days of pregnancy, but forbids abortion on demand. If it is to happen, serious and stringent conditions must be met, as when the fetus represents a danger to the life of the mother.[38] In addition, it can happen that the medical good of the patient might serve the patient's perception of the good, as when she asks for an abortion, but does not meet the spiritual good as Pellegrino portrays it, which is the higher level of good, nor does it honor the moral absolutes that Pellegrino holds on to so firmly. The four levels of the good are bound to conflict because moral life is complex as are the cases that physicians face. Moral absolutes exist, but they alone cannot guide the decisions of physicians dealing with such complexities because exceptions and grey zones very often occur.

1.7. Moral Absolutes

In his article "Some Things Ought Never Be Done," Pellegrino argues that there exist in the nature of the physician-patient relationship certain moral absolutes which are essential to the realization of the good of the patient (the good of the patient being the end of this relationship) (2005a). These moral absolutes derive from the principle of doing good and avoiding evil. But how can we have a clinical encounter bound by moral absolutes when the definition of medicine is a function of the good of the patient as the patient perceives it? It is an empirical fact that some patients' perceptions of their good often disregard if not disagree with these subsidiary absolutes, as when patients seek abortions, or they want to have their lives terminated when they are in unbearable pain or when medical treatment is futile,

---

38. The moral status of the fetus (concerning such questions as whether or not the fetus is a person with the rights that belong to persons, including the right to life) is a central issue in the debate concerning the morality of abortion.

or they refuse life-saving measures,[39] and at times they want to be lied to.[40] If we are to accept Pellegrino's moral absolutes as overriding, as elements of an absolutist deontology, the conclusion will be that the physician will not be able to serve the patient's good as he sees it if the patient sees his good as being in opposition to the absolutes Pellegrino presents. Individual perceptions can only accidentally fit with absolute claims and so too with the needs of the patient. However, Pellegrino himself notes that the patient's preferences are not paramount nor absolute since to take them as such would be to "violate the autonomy of the physician[41] and would also amount to asking the physician to lay aside his own moral integrity and to become *value neutral*," which, according to Pellegrino, is a "psychological impossibility" (2001a, 572). In a letter to the author, Pellegrino states that in case the physician's conception of the good is different from that of the patient at each of the four levels, except in extreme emergency, he would not breach the patient's concept of the good even if that conception disagreed with any of the four levels of the good.[42] Yet, this does not mean that he must cooperate and do what the patient wishes. One can also, *à la rigueur*, argue that the four different kinds of good offered by Pellegrino can come into conflict. Consider a patient with diabetes: his medical good would be to treat his diabetes and emphasize the need to eat regularly, in small portions, certain kinds of food. His spiritual good however might be that he fast during certain assigned religious days, which might negatively impact his health. If the spiritual good supersedes the medical good, what ought the physician to do when the patient presents to him while fasting, complaining of a sudden onset of his disease? Another example would be when a Jehovah's Witness refuses blood transfusions. Here, we have a conflict between the medical good and the human good on the one hand, and the perceptions of the patient and the spiritual good on the other. It is a fact that doctors and patients can differ in their perceptions of what makes for human flourishing. Pellegrino's view sheds light on the fact that doctors and patients do differ on what they think of the good, and how they can differ and at what levels.

---

39. Like the case of a patient who is a Jehovah's Witness and refuses a life-saving blood transfusion. Pellegrino argues that the patient's spiritual good is the highest good that should be served. Aborting a genetically impaired fetus or discontinuing life support cannot be considered healing acts since they violate that highest good (2001a, 571). Yet, it can be argued that many religions nowadays argue for the opposite. Hence the tension between the patient's perception of his good and the moral absolutes that the physician is supposed to follow in order to be a good physician following the ends of medicine. Still, it is important to note that Pellegrino's conception of the patient's good is not thoroughly subjective as it precedes non-maleficence, for to him and Thomasma (1993), the first principle of medical ethics is to act for the benefit of the patient and if one does that, one *ipso facto* avoids harm.

40. To a letter the author sent to him in October 2010 inquiring about whether he expects relativists to agree with him, Pellegrino responded, "I certainly do not expect the relativists to agree with me. The very use of the term "absolute" excludes that. In the case of abortion, assisted suicide, and the use of embryonic stem cells, I see no room for compromise. I cannot morally expect others to comply with my absolutes or impose my concepts by violent means. But, neither can they ask me to violate my conscience." (Personal Communication, 18 October 2010).

41. The patient will then have to find another physician with sympathetic views.

42. Pellegrino, personal communication, 18 October 2010.

Yet to him:

> *[T]he end of medicine is the good. That is what is absolute, but the perceptions, conceptions of that good may be mistaken. The physician is not empowered to override the patient's conception. On the other hand, the patient, simply on the basis of his perception of the good, . . . cannot demand that the physician do what he thinks evil.*[43]

Ultimately, and in case of a conflict of perceptions concerning what constitutes the good, no one has precedence over the other, and the autonomy of each is safeguarded. If the patient were to impose his vision of the good on the physician, the latter would perhaps would not be able to live with herself and her profession any longer, experiencing a dissociation between professional and personal conscience; and if the physician were to impose her conception of the good, the patient who sees the situation otherwise would be unhappy. If there are things that ought never be done, what is the good physician to do in this case? Ought the duties attached to the role of the physician be absolute in nature rather than prima facie? If *good* is tied to *end*, and if a good physician is one who performs her function well by exhibiting well the ends of medicine, then the good physician in this case may have to break the absolutes of medicine and perform medicine situationally in an Aristotelian fashion using her *phronesis*.[44] But did not Aristotle himself speak of things that ought never be done although his ethics is viewed as a situational one? Another question that arises is: what happens in cases where Pellegrino's absolutes come into conflict? Although Pellegrino argues that it is in the nature of the moral absolutes not to conflict,[45] one can imagine a situation where the medical good of the patient lies in her aborting a fetus, as in the example mentioned above, or situations when breaking one's promises, depending on the situation, is the morally right thing to do, where protecting the dignity of the patient might lead to the physician foregoing an extraordinary attempt at keeping the patient alive. Consider the example of euthanasia: does a patient's right to die entail a physician's duty to kill? The question to begin with is about the patient's right to die, which, merits a lot of discussion but which falls beyond the scope of this book. Yet, for the sake of argument, it will

---

43. Pellegrino, personal communication, 13 May 2010.

44. At times, a doctor will have to perform an abortion to save the life of the mother. Yet, in a situation where the mother is a criminal sentenced to death and the court order is final and she will be executed in a few days, it is only normal for the physician to save the life of the baby in a situation in which only one will live. Here the moral absolutes are violated, and it would be immoral not to violate them.

45. In an email, dated 13 May 2010, to the author of this book, Pellegrino commented that "it is in the nature of a moral absolute that it is binding in all situations. (...) Moral absolutes are not like the four principles that can conflict with each other."

be said that to some, like Pellegrino, the physician's duty never to kill is inviolable and paramount, while for others, the duty to relieve suffering might outweigh it. Nevertheless, for this duty to be inviolable means that it is unconditionally morally binding. This is perhaps a bit too Kantian for the contemporary virtue ethicist that Pellegrino is. Given the complexities of modern medical conditions, can physicians really have any duties of this kind? I am not contesting that doctors have a duty not to kill, but I am merely looking at the unconditionality of this duty, particularly for a thinker who stresses the autonomy of the patient, the importance of the patient's view of his good, and beneficence as being a primary end of medicine. The duty of the physician here is to provide that patient with whatever will benefit him. But when medical treatment is futile, when the dying patient is increasingly suffering with no hope of a cure, in what sense can one argue that keeping that patient alive benefits him? Is not this blind obedience to rules detrimental to the profession and in contradiction with the spirit of the *phronimos*,[46] who has his eyes on many things at the same time, like the wise steersman in charge of a ship in a stormy weather? Would the benefit to the patient and his family not be a quick and painless death if, all things considered, this is the wish of the patient? Medicine is based on the patient's right to life. When the patient renounces this right, the physician cannot force it upon him. Pellegrino argues that euthanasia undermines the trust that exists between physician and patient. To him, when euthanasia is considered, "this trust relationship is seriously distorted. Healing now includes killing. . . . How can patients trust that the doctor will pursue every effective and beneficent measure when she can relieve herself of a difficult challenge by influencing the patient to choose death?" (1992, 98). Questions that arise at this point include: what is *included* in that trust? Does the patient trust the physician never to cause his death, or to respect his wishes and values regarding his healthcare choices, or to do what is best for him? Would the patient feel that his trust has been betrayed and his wishes disrespected and ignored when his physician keeps him in agony, against his wishes, on a life-sustaining machine, dying slowly when he could, by a simple act of unplugging, put an end to his misery? Can the physician be trusted to use her *phronesis* and decide which acts of euthanasia are morally justified and which are not? This is not to say that there is no risk of a slippery slope, which is another issue altogether. By stating that there are certain things that ought never be done, including euthanasia and abortion, Pellegrino is too rigid in his absolutism. The only absolute is the fact that the end of medicine is to give care and cure where possible. In order to do that, at times the

---

46. According to Aristotle, a *phronimos* is a wise resource.

physician will have to break the moral absolutes to which Pellegrino so adamantly adheres. Does Pellegrino assume that the physician already agrees to his moral absolutes and does not agree to what may be called the patient's "unconventional" view of his good? We are witnessing an era when medical students are voicing their concern about taking the Hippocratic oath precisely because of its absolutism. Pellegrino is aware of this but is also aware that: "The Hippocratic oath has been in a parlous state, especially in the past three decades, since the rise of contemporary bioethics" (2002a, 99).[47] Yet he continues to argue that "perhaps for many the medical oath is today a shard of a fractured ancient image. But enough of that image remains in the consciousness of the profession to remind us that to forget it entirely would be to make medicine a commercial, industrial or proletarian enterprise" (2002a, 99). The Hippocratic oath, as well as other oaths, exist to remind medical practitioners of the internal ends of medicine. The question that arises at this point is whether these ends are universal or whether they are a function of particular times and places.

1.8. The Importance of Trust in the Physician-Patient Relationship

Medicine is a human activity, not a purely scientific skill. It is a profession that is actualized during encounters between patients and physicians, and its goal is predominantly the good of the patient. The physician, by virtue of her profession, should have no other good in mind. This is what compels the patient to trust the physician in the hope that she will restore some of the patient's lost autonomy and pride and will do her best to heal him. In other words, the patient trusts that the physician will serve the ends of medicine. As Pellegrino puts it, "[t]rust is most problematic when we are in states of special dependence—in illness, old age, or infancy, or when we are in need of healing" (Pellegrino and Thomasma 1993, 65). In what follows, I argue that trust is a quintessential ingredient of the physician-patient relationship, and that trusting the physician entails not only a trust in the system which gave the physician the education and license but also trust in the character of the physician—trust that she will not abuse her power, but will do whatever is within that power to heal the patient. For this reason, it is important to cultivate physicians of fine moral fiber who will serve the ends of medicine as they ought to be served.

---

47. In 2006, Pellegrino stated that "[t]he great canon of medical morality, the Hippocratic Oath, is being honored more in the breach than in observance. Each one of its prescriptions has been questioned by some physicians and believed by others." (2006, 66).

Trust affects and cements the moral relationship between patient and physician. The personal values of the physician could be external to the ends of medicine. Her values could be governed by self-interest and greed, and if this were the case, the physician could not serve the internal ends of medicine. One can also add to this the fact that trust can be abused,[48] particularly since the patient qua patient is placed in a relationship in which he is forced to trust the physician with his health. In the medical encounter, trust is valued for what it helps to bring about; it is beyond technical expertise and is the essence of the medical encounter. Without this element to the encounter, there is no medicine to be practiced and the ends of medicine will not be served as they ought to be since the patient might not reveal the intimacies of his psyche or even illness to the physician out of fear that the information might be abused.[49] According to Pellegrino, trust is "ineradicable" and "we need the help of doctors to surmount or cope with our most pressing human needs. We must depend on their fidelity to trust and their desire to protect rather than exploit our vulnerability" (Pellegrino and Thomasma 1993, 65). After all, the physician-patient relationship, at the very heart of medicine, is built on trust, and hence the physician needs to be trustworthy, someone virtuous enough not to abuse the information she has been given by the patient. Reflecting on trust, Pellegrino contends that trust in the medical profession has drastically deteriorated and that patients view physicians as being more interested in money than in their patients' well-being; physicians sometimes are viewed as exploiters, rather than guardians, of medical knowledge (Pellegrino and Thomasma 1993, 65–78). When physicians overlook the ends of medicine and concentrate on personal values, self-interest, and greed—when they yield to marketplace forces, and view the patient as a client instead of a patient—then they lose sight of its moral dimension, the practice of medicine is distorted, and harm ensues. The physician-patient relationship is essentially fiduciary, which makes the bond of trust vital for the diagnostic and therapeutic processes. As Pellegrino and Thomasma have pointed out, "the end of medicine, its justifying principle, is, in the final analysis, a moral one: the "good" of a person seeking help. The choice of what ought to be done turns on questions of value, morality, and interpersonal dynamics. These questions can be studied scientifically, to be sure, but they cannot be defined by scientific considerations alone" (1981, 147). The phrase "good of the patient" refers to both his physical and psychological good. Francis Peabody's exhortation summarizes the key elements of the physician-patient relationship:

---

48. The vulnerability of patients can be abused for profit or power. As Pellegrino and Thomasma put it, "[t]o trust and entrust is to become vulnerable and dependent on the good will and motivations of those we trust" (2003, 65).

49. One of the main critiques against what has come to be known as internet medicine is the absence of the clinical encounter and the requisite physician-patient relationship.

The good physician knows his patients through and through, and his knowledge is bought dearly. Time, sympathy, and understanding must be lavishly dispensed, but the reward is to be found in that personal bond which forms the greatest satisfaction of the practice of medicine. One of the essential qualities of the clinician is interest in humanity, for the secret of the care of the patient is in caring for the patient. (Peabody 1927, 818)

In the physician-patient encounter, trust is essential. It has instrumental value, as it upholds a fractured autonomy, increases cooperation, enhances treatment which is based on correct information, builds a healthy relationship that is vital for both patient and physician, and is crucial to the success of the entire diagnosis-prognosis-treatment triad. It is intrinsic to the notion of trust that one has faith in the good will of the one trusted to do what is best for the person doing the trusting. In "Trust and Anti-Trust," Annette Baier defines trust by referring to the expectation of the one trusting to benefit from the good will of the trusted. She speaks of "intentional trusting" which "require[s] awareness of one's confidence that the trusted will not harm one, although they can" (1986, 235). Baier continues to say that often we need the help of the trusted in "looking after the things we most value, so we have no choice but to allow some others to be in a position to harm them" (1986, 236). What is it that human beings value most? Health is one of those things, and we entrust it to physicians, believing in their good will not to harm one of our most valued goods. Baier continues:

Where one depends on another's good will, one is necessarily vulnerable to the limits of that good will. One leaves others an opportunity to harm one when one trusts, and also shows one's confidence that they will not take it. Reasonable trust will require good grounds for such confidence in another's good will, or at least the absence of good grounds for expecting their ill will or indifference (1986, 235).

This applies especially when the trusted is the physician and the one trusting is the patient who expects to benefit from the former's good will as long as the affiliation continues to exist. This ties in quite well with the universal characteristics of the ends of medicine. To my knowledge, patients around the world build their relationships with their physicians on the assumption that they can trust them with their health and privacy. The problem arises when physicians of less than trustworthy character deceive patients and work for their self-interests instead of the good of the patient. Examples abound and include physicians who do not refer patients to specialists, but continue treating them, dragging them to their clinic more than necessary although the ailment is not in their area of specialty; physicians who ask patients to undergo a number of useless tests for personal gain; physicians who are prey to conflict of interest and do not declare this to their patients; and surgeons who do not tell their patients that what they suffer from can be resolved by non-invasive procedures. If the physician uses the information that the patient gives her for purposes other than his good and if the physician abuses the power that she has and does not honor the ends of medicine, trust will fail, and with it the entire physician-patient relationship cemented by this trust. Patients do not worry, or at least, should not worry, about the motives of physicians when they visit them or disclose information. Their doctors are their advocates, and to act any differently would be to betray that trust, to break the relationship, and to use the profession of medicine for other than its legitimate ends.[50] A major guarantee for remaining true to the values of the profession and the ends of medicine is the possession of good character, and it is the role of medical schools to cultivate such character in the neophyte student of medicine. In medicine, the moral and the technical cannot be divorced, or else medicine becomes schizophrenic, and the practice of medicine will witness its own demise.

Michael Stocker attempted to show that "not to be moved by what one values—what one believes good, nice, right, beautiful, and so on—bespeaks a malady of the spirit" (1976, 454). He argues that such persons will unavoidably experience a gap between their values and motives which will lead to moral schizophrenia. Thus, since modern ethical theories result in this malady, they are gravely defective. Regardless of whether Stocker was right in saying that such moral theories are flawed because they result in a malady of the spirit, it remains a fact that a gap between values and motives will have dramatic effects in a profession like medicine. One might argue that as long as the actions of a physician are in accord with what she should do, then it does not matter what her motives are; I beg to differ. If a person's morality and motives are different, there is no guarantee that this person will continue to behave in accordance with morality, that he will *do the right thing even when no one is looking*. When physicians suffer a disharmony between acts and motives, a malady of the spirit and the intellect ensues. When they have not internalized the virtues, and they act morally because they are afraid of sanctions, seek promotions, someone is in the room watching them, or want rewards, they are schizophrenic in Stocker's sense, and will suffer instances of weakness of will. Thus, virtues are essential for the making of

---

50. A patient who feels that he cannot trust his physician will not be able to benefit from the clinical encounter to the full. In such encounters, the ends of medicine will not be met, and the physician will fail to do her duty.

the good physician who will not falter nor be lured by the external ends of medicine. Consequently, medical schools need to educate students of medicine in the virtues[51] and help them internalize those virtues in such a way that those virtues become second nature to students. When virtues are not internalized, when the character of the physician is not solid, the ends of medicine become blurred and physicians falter. That it happened with Aesculapius, the god of medicine, is significant. Pindar's myth portrays the son of Apollo lured by "the love of gain" and "enthralled by a splendid fee of gold displayed upon the palm" (Pindar 1924, 191). Examples of physicians who request unnecessary invasive procedures to increase their reimbursement, request redundant tests to supplement their income, admit patients to the hospital unnecessarily, use them as subjects in clinical trials without their consent, or fall victim to conflicts of interest as an upshot of the endowment they accept from the pharmaceutical industry are not anecdotal. In this manner, some physicians abuse the power they have by virtue of being healers.

Another attribute of the physician-patient encounter is an imbalance of power between the trusting (patient) and the trusted (physician). On the one hand, we have a vulnerable patient with reduced autonomy, and on the other an expert who can offer medical care. This vulnerability compels the patient to trust physicians, more so when the sickness is grave and the physician is seen as a shaman in a white coat, a deliverer who will save the patient. Physician and philosopher Howard Brody spoke of "power" as being central to the relationship between physician and patient since physicians, owing to their position, have considerable power to alter the course of illness. He proposes three kinds of power possessed by physicians:

Aesculapian, charismatic, and social. The physician by virtue of her education in medicine, possesses Aesculapian power. It is an "impersonal power, it is transferable from any physician to any other of comparable skill and experience" (Brody 1992, 16). Charismatic power cannot be transferred in that it is based on the personal qualities of the physician. Such qualities include being decisive, courageous, firm, and kind. Social power comes about as a result of the social status of the physician. According to Brody, it is "axiomatic that the use of power must go hand in hand with its potential misuse" (1992, 20), and he concludes that the main ethical problem that medicine has to face is how to use this power responsibly (1992, 36). Brody maintains that "this same power can, with only subtle redirection, be used against the patient's behalf. The problem is to empower physicians for the performance

---

51. This will be tackled in chapters two and three.

of their essential tasks while protecting the patient from the potential misuse and abuses of power" (1992, 36). The physician is trusted with "discretionary powers," to use Baier's term, but the patient assumes—rightly, by virtue of what the word profession means—that the physician will not abuse these powers for the good of anyone or anything other than the patient. This relates again to the ends of medicine, what a physician professes to be, and finally to the importance of bringing up physicians with good character. This, after all, was the predicament of Tolstoy's Ivan Ilyich: he went to a physician entrusting him with his health but was faced with a character that inspired distrust and service to something other than the ends of medicine, which explains his tragedy as a patient.

In this chapter I have established that medicine is a moral enterprise based on the covenant of trust that forms the heart of the clinical encounter. I have presented some of Edmund Pellegrino's basic ideas about the ends of medicine being internal to the profession as opposed to external. I also presented some of his ideas relating to the philosophy of medicine and provided arguments about some issues that he raises in relation to the good of the patient and moral absolutes. I have argued that virtues are vital for the making of a good physician and need to be internalized if the ends of medicine, as portrayed by Pellegrino, are to be met. It is my contention that the function of a physician is tied to the ends of medicine. The nature of medicine as a moral endeavor renders this function different from the function of, say, a salesman or a craftsman. For each of these vocations, the telos is different and, quoting Aristotle in the opening of his *Nicomachean Ethics*: "Every art and every inquiry, and similarly every action and pursuit, is thought to aim at some good; and for this reason the good has rightly been declared to be that at which all things aim" (1947, 307). In medicine, the *telos* is the good of the patient and the physician has to be equipped with certain virtues that make "a man good and which makes him do his own work well" (1947, 338). This has not been difficult to achieve throughout history, and the traditional physician, as portrayed in the 1927 painting *The Doctor* by Sir Samuel Luke Fildes, seemed to encompass the old image of the virtuous physician. Yet, there has emerged a new paradigm where being virtuous and good are considered to be synonymous with being a simpleton and weak. This moral change arose from several sources, mostly the same ones that led to the de-professionalization of modern medicine. Thus, what is needed is a new paradigm shift. Education paves the way for the smooth emergence of a new/old paradigm so that it will not be rejected in an era when medicine is once again seen as the privilege of crude scientists. Therefore, the fundamental question becomes: how can we bring about a physician who demonstrates the character traits that prompt her to act well and in accordance with the ends of medicine?

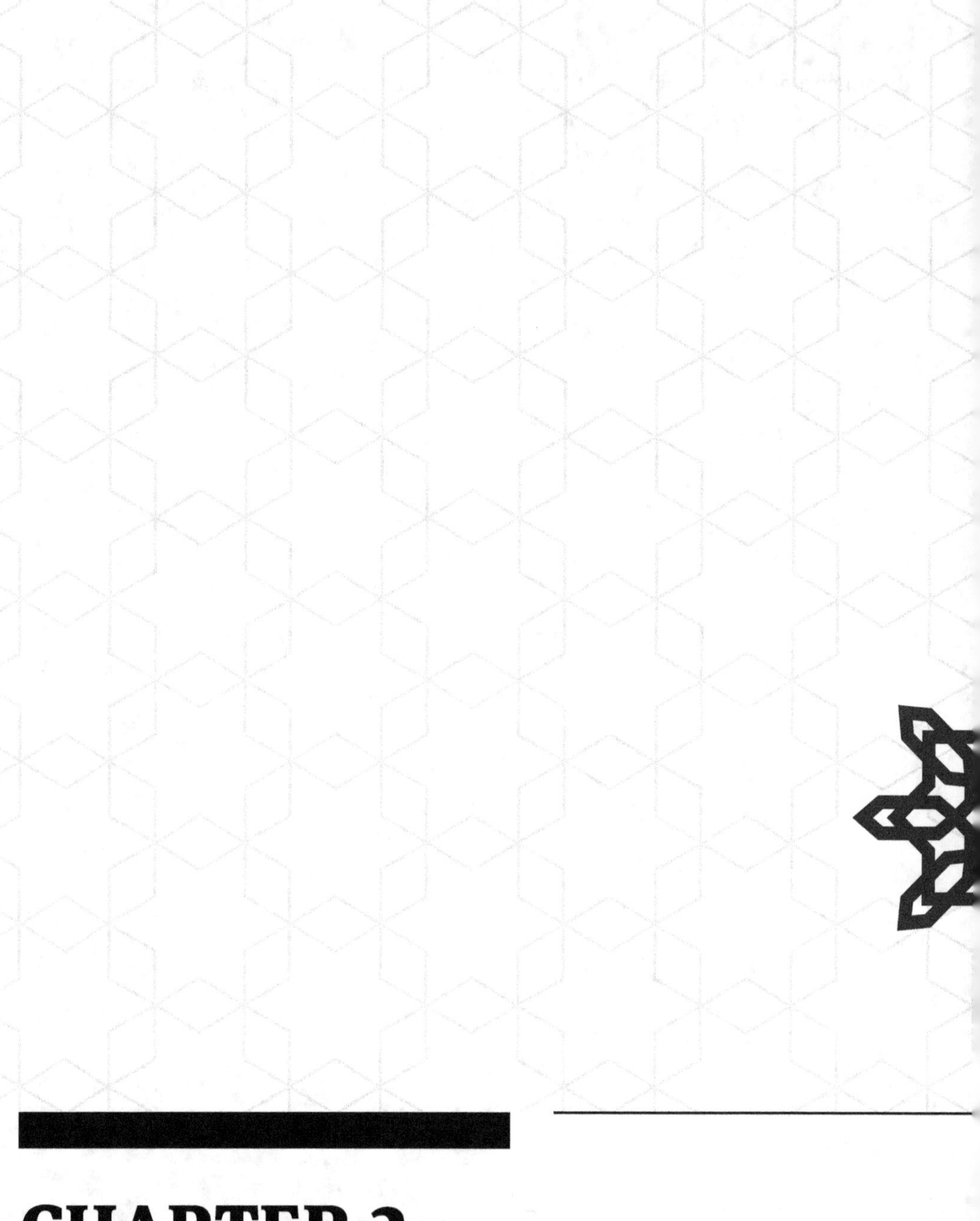

CHAPTER 2:
ARISTOTLE'S VIRTUE ETHICS AND THE PROFESSION OF MEDICINE

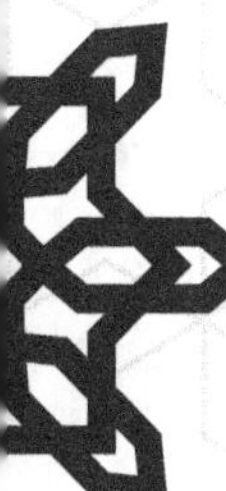

Must we agree with Socrates that compassion
in a medical graduate is a "gift from the gods"?
I think not.

—G. Pence, "Can compassion be taught?"
(1983, 190)

There is a revival of interest in virtual ethics among scholars of modern moral philosophy, in general, and medical ethics, in particular, and Aristotle is considered its finest advocate. His concern was mainly with "what kind of person one ought to become," whereas the concern of moral theories such as deontology and utilitarianism is primarily with "what is the right action." For this reason, virtue ethics is often referred to as "character ethics," the central notion being that of developing the right character. For Aristotle, ethics had a practical aim: to do good and act well; hence, his emphasis on *praxis*. A person does the right thing not because he is following a certain set of rules or out of respect for a certain principle, but rather, as a result of possessing the right virtues. In chapter one, I argued that medicine is a moral endeavor and that good character is fundamental to the making of a good physician who should live up to her profession and serve the ends of medicine, which are universal and internal to the profession. I also argued that virtues are vital to the making of a good physician. In this chapter, I will begin by presenting a brief account of Aristotle's virtue ethics and how the habitual performing of virtuous action will eventually induce a person to acquire the virtues. I will then move on to discuss the role that Aristotle's ethics can play in the moral development of medical students during their years of training in medical school, and I argue that virtue ethics can help in the making of the good physician. Since one might wonder why I have chosen virtue ethics and not deontology or utilitarianism, I will first tackle this issue, albeit briefly, and then discuss the inevitable question of whether the virtues can be taught.

Virtues are dispositions in a person's character that prompt him to act in a particular way. Applied to medicine, we can say that what motivates the actions of a physician is her character. Hence, virtues have an important role to play in the ethical conduct of a person. So, what is virtue and how is it acquired?

A brief account of Aristotle's virtue ethics, as presented in his *Nichomachean* Ethics (hereafter, *NE*), is indispensable in order to answer these questions. Aristotle opens his *NE* by stating that everything we do aims towards some good, and that every action has a goal for the sake of which we act. Thus, "the good has rightly been declared to be that at which all things aim" (1947, 308). This, good, he argues, is the chief good which is "always desirable in itself and never for the sake of something else" (1947, 317). This chief good, we are later told, is *eudaimonia*, usually translated as happiness or human flourishing. Furthermore, Aristotle maintained that what human beings should do or how they should behave is contained in their very nature, just like the acorn has in it the potential of developing into an oak. Thus, when human beings develop as they ought to develop, they flourish and become happy: "Pleasure completes this activity . . . as an end which supervenes as the bloom of youth does on those in the flower of their age" (1947, 526). The opposite is equally true. A heart that pumps blood well is, in that sense, a happy heart, while one that is ailing and does not perform its function well is not. The notion of a "function" is central to Aristotle's philosophy of human flourishing, for "the good and the well is thought to reside in the function" (1947, 318).

According to Aristotle, everything has a function. The function of a knife is to cut, and the function of a heart is to pump blood. However, since the human soul is distinctive in its capacity for reason (the appetitive and vegetative parts we share with other organisms), the function of human beings is to live an active life in accordance with reason. Furthermore, Aristotle says that "the virtue of man also will be the state of character which makes a man good and which makes him do his own work well"[1] (1947, 338). Thus, the notion of virtue is tied to the notion of function and the highest good (*eudaimonia*), which is chosen for its own sake: "Virtue, then, is a state of character concerned with choice, lying in a mean, i.e., the mean relative to us, this being determined by a rational principle, and by that principle by which the man of practical wisdom would determine it" (1947, 340). A person possessing virtues will eventually act in accordance with them and will even reach a state of inner happiness since happiness is an activity of the soul in accordance with virtue. The virtues that the person develops will, with time, become "second nature" and develop into character traits akin to congenital dispositions that are reliable and stable. Equipped with these traits, a person can be relied upon to act dependably over time. In Book One of his *NE*, Aristotle argues that the chief good is a life that is peculiarly human. The good proper to man, a rational activity in accordance with virtue, can be understood as intellectual virtue (e.g., wisdom) or moral virtue (e.g., honesty). What does a virtuous activity consist of and how are virtues acquired?

---

1. Unlike his teacher Plato, who believed in one Good in the world of Forms, Aristotle believed that everything has its own good (animals, plants, humans). This good is defined by examining the nature of the entity in question. The nature of that entity is, in turn, understood by looking at its function.

2.1. Virtuous Activity and the Acquisition of Virtues

Consider the following scenario: you are walking down the street and you see a beggar whom you know to be needy and sick. You have always walked by him and you have never been charitable to him although you have always had more than enough money on you. On that particular Tuesday morning, as you were walking with people with whom you are trying to do business, you give him money, making sure that your partners see your act of benevolence, hoping their view of you as a charitable and good person might positively affect the course of your business with them. Aristotle would argue that this is not a virtuous act since generosity and benevolence are virtues precisely because of the *reason* for which charity was given. Thus, a person's action is directly related to the virtues of that person and to his character. Had you given money to the needy beggar because you were a charitable, benevolent person by character, the situation would have been different. Thus, unlike the outcome of the arts, the important thing is not merely the act that was done, but *how* it was done. The worth of a virtuous act is in attaining a virtuous character. Aristotle put forward three conditions that must be met for an act to be considered virtuous: "The agent also must be in a certain condition when he does them; in the first place, he must have knowledge; second, he must choose the acts and choose them for their own sake; and third, his action must proceed from a firm and unchangeable character" (1947, 336). Virtuous activity is such that it implies the acknowledgment of and acquiescence to an ideal of human excellence that leads one to what is noble (Greek: *kalon*). Thus, in the example above, the benevolent person should choose benevolence because benevolence is noble and contributes to human flourishing (although not in the sense of being a means to an end since a flourishing life consists of virtuous activity). This brings us back to the notion of *praxis,* a peculiarly human activity that pushes one towards what is noble and worthwhile. Since happiness consists in virtuous activity, the central question becomes: how does one become virtuous?

Aristotle is renowned for his view that virtues and vices arise through habituation: "[M]oral virtue comes about as a result of habit" (1947, 331). According to him, we acquire our virtues and our vices just as we acquire arts and crafts—through a process of learning marked by repetition and habituation: "[T]he virtues we get by first exercising them, as also happens in the case of the arts as well. For the things we have to learn before we can do them, we learn by doing them; e.g., men become builders by building and lyre players by playing the lyre; so too we become just by doing just acts, temperate by doing temperate acts, brave by doing brave acts" (1947, 331). Thus, a physician who deals inhumanely with patients will acquire the habit of inhumane dealing and becomes an inhumane physician. To become a humane physician, she must break her old habits and acquire new habits of humaneness. An important point in Aristotle's philosophy of education has to do with the fact that human beings cannot learn something that is contrary to their nature, "for nothing that exists by nature can form a habit contrary to its nature. For instance, the stone which by nature moves downwards cannot be habituated to move upwards, not even if one tries to train it by throwing it up ten thousand times; nor can fire be habituated to move downwards, nor can anything else that by nature behaves in one way be trained to behave in another. Neither by nature, then, nor contrary to nature do the virtues arise in us; rather we are adapted by nature to receive them, and are made perfect by habit" (1947, 331). Aristotle also contends that "it makes no small difference, then, whether we form habits of one kind or of another from our very youth; it makes a very great difference, or rather *all* the difference" (1947, 332).[2] Ultimately, habits become second nature. They can be unlearned but it is not a quick or easy process. To learn good habits and unlearn bad ones, proper training is needed. However, this cannot be done alone, as one needs the guidance of a teacher, a role model, or a mentor, so to speak; such teachers should be virtuous persons themselves. The virtuous teacher possesses the necessary wisdom to guide others and is a role model to emulate.[3] Ultimately, the learner will learn to do the virtuous activity for its own sake; he will be keen on engaging in it because it is noble.

The heart of Aristotle's account of moral virtues lies in his doctrine of the mean. Thus, virtue is a mean lying between excess and deficiency; courage is a mean between cowardice and rashness; modesty is a mean between shamelessness and bashfulness. The mean, according to Aristotle, cannot be measured mathematically, and indeed, there is no miraculous formula or a magical moral calculator to help make the right decisions. This is why "it is no easy task to be good. For in everything, it is no easy task to find the middle; e.g., to find the middle of a circle is not for everyone but for him who knows; . . . but to do this to the right person, to the right extent, at the right time, with the right motive, and in the right way, that is not for everyone, nor is it easy; wherefore goodness is both rare and laudable and noble"

---

2. Italics in the original. Thus, the double challenge in medical school is to help medical students unlearn bad habits and learn good ones. Is there enough time to do this? How can this be assessed? These issues will be considered in chapter four.

3. One question that arises at this point is the following: to learn good habits and unlearn bad ones, one should (among other things) have a good teacher, a role model. What about the first teacher or role model (let us call this the problem of the first generation), how did he acquire the virtues in the absence of a first wise teacher? Did he just emerge?

(1947, 346). All moral virtues are about passions and actions, and they allow "excess, defect, and the intermediate" (1947, 339). Virtue is a type of mean, since "it aims at what is intermediate" (1947, 340), the intermediate being that which is suitable to the particular situation. For example, speaking of certain passions and emotions, Aristotle states: "to feel them at the right time, with reference to the right objects, towards the right people, with the right motive, and in the right way, is what is both intermediate and best, and this is characteristic of virtue" (1947, 340). Ultimately, he summarizes his view of the virtues by stating that "virtue, then, is a state of character concerned with choice, lying in a mean, i.e., the mean relative to us, this being determined by a rational principle, and by that principle by which the man of practical wisdom would determine it" (1947, 340). Practical wisdom (*phronesis*) is the new and very important crowning characteristic (the art of practical judgment) that Aristotle introduces here. *Phronesis*, the capacity to think about practical matters, allows for deliberation and judgment in difficult moral situations. Practical wisdom, Aristotle tells us "is the quality of mind concerned with things just and noble and good for man" (1947, 438). In it, intellectual and moral virtues are united and the *phronimos* can see the right thing to be done, for "moral virtue makes us aim at the right mark, and practical wisdom makes us take the right means" (1947, 439). It involves a blend of understanding and experience and consists of the capability to deal appropriately with specific situations. Thus, a person of practical wisdom draws on previous experience and is continuously enhancing his understanding in light of the specific situations with which he is faced.

2.2. Aristotelian Ethics and the Medical School

William Osler was one of the physicians who insisted on the importance of good character in the neophyte physician and stressed the importance of educating the heart in addition to the mind (Osler 1932). Along the same lines, Howard Brody cautions against treating patients as chunks of meat transported from one part of the hospital to another (Brody 1992). Patients are human beings with a past, a present, and a future. They carry the weight of their illnesses and their damaged autonomy and injured dignity with them. These are even more compromised by having to succumb to a relationship of power imbalance that makes it essential that the physician behave in a certain way. The physician has to be a *certain kind* of person, one that a businessman, a hairdresser, or shoemaker need not be. What mechanism is there that guarantees the making of such a physician? To begin with, education plays a major role in the making of physicians. One can argue that the purpose of medical education is not only to produce a physician, but a certain kind of physician. The medical curriculum is said to be designed to achieve these goals, and medical faculties across the world have mission statements with a section about the moral education of students. For example, the mission statement of the Yale University School of Medicine states that students of medicine should be "committed to serving others and devoted to the care of their patients. They must bring intention and action as well as empathy and compassion to the doctor-patient relationship. They must demonstrate honesty and integrity in all of their professional interactions." The Johns Hopkins University mission statement states that graduates will "[d]isplay the personal attributes of compassion, honesty and integrity in relationship with patients, families, and the medical community," and that of the American University of Beirut Faculty of Medicine speaks of "a strong commitment of the faculty to educate young men and women to become excellent physicians with humane and high ethical standards, as well as technical expertise." The learning objectives for medical student education of the Association of American Medical Colleges state that physicians must be altruistic, honest, compassionate, and respectful (Anderson et al. 1998). Mission statements are public promises and open declarations. Thus, schools are and ought to be held responsible for those statements. Hence, the question that arises is: how can medical schools live up to these mission statements and educate students of medicine to grow into upright doctors? Here, it is my contention that Aristotle's virtue ethics becomes relevant, for when we speak of "compassion," "empathy," "honesty," "humane physicians," "ethical standards," and other similar traits, we are referring to habits and attitudes, not to matters of knowledge. Desired student outcomes (in our case, those of the medical student) cannot be sought outside the realm of character. First, what is so particular about the medical student, the doctor-to-be, that makes it vital to worry about his character (which is not the case, perhaps, of the novice shoemaker)?

Medical students are on the way to becoming physicians, to joining a profession that has a special significance. This is precisely why the student of medicine is made to take an oath upon graduation, and it is this oath, not the medical degree, that imposes on him a commitment to a certain manner of life that the shoemaker or the hairdresser is not obliged to follow.[4] The oath is an assertion that strengthens the physician's determination to behave with integrity in times of conflict and weakness.

---

4. There are other professions whose members take oaths, like lawyers, nurses, and some educators. In that sense, they do have some moral *oughts* by which they have to abide.

As stated by Pellegrino, "without the Oath the doctor is a skilled technician or laborer whose knowledge fits him for an occupation but not a profession" (2002b, 379). This oath is, in so many ways, a commitment to a way of life. According to Albert Jonsen, Galen spoke of the medical student as one whose life is shaped by temperance and justice, and who lives by other virtues as well (Jonsen 2000, 10). Galen's sense of ethics stresses mainly the character of the physician, emphasizing virtues rather than duties and rules (Jonsen 2000, 11). People who take an oath are oriented towards a certain way of life and, as Daniel Sulmasy says, "swear to be certain kinds of persons" (2006, 96). Therefore, as Sulmasy continues, "the ethics of an oath ought to be the ethics of virtue" (2006, 96) and this ethics "points to a transcendental ideal (toward moral perfection) and demands a sincere effort to strive towards that ideal." (2006, 97) Thus, the good physician is the one who, in addition to being skilled, also possesses certain character traits. There is a need for such character traits precisely because of the nature of the medical profession, which is closely tied to the ends of medicine as described in chapter one. How does one ensure that students of medicine will develop into the physicians characterized in the different mission statements of medical schools? Put differently, how does one ensure that these potential physicians will possess the character necessary for them to be good physicians?

2.3. Virtue Ethics and the Good Physician

Virtue ethics has witnessed a rebirth in modern-day thought, particularly as reflected in Elizabeth Anscombe's "Modern Moral Philosophy" (1958) and Alasdair MacIntyre's *After Virtue* (1984). A major strength of virtue theory derives from the fact that it concentrates on developing the character of the agent instead of relying on rules, and thus does not rely on notions of moral obligation per se.[5] Relying on moral obligations does not give the guarantee of consistency in good deeds that, arguably, virtue ethics offers as a result of developing a virtuous character. One question that arises at this point is: why cite Aristotle and not Michael Slote or someone else, for that matter? My answer is simple and straightforward: Slote, whose agent-based philosophy is moral sentimentalism, offers a theory about morality by which empathy, which he labels the "cement of morality" (Slote 2010, 27), can be conveyed to children through induction and modeling, drawing on the work of psychologist Martin Hoffman. Slote does not put forward a full theory of

---

5. Such notions, argues Anscombe, are based on theological background assumptions that do not hold any longer. Why virtue ethics, and not deontology or utilitarianism, for example, is an issue I will come to shortly.

moral education that can guide us into graduating virtuous physicians, presuming instead a sentimentalist standpoint of morality which "rests on the idea that being moral amounts to being (fully) empathically caring *vis-à-vis* others" (Slote 2013, 31). He assumes that empathy exists but needs to be nurtured. However, we are not told how, if at all, it can really be nurtured in adults (which is crucial for our project). He argues that empathy arises in a normal way against the background of self-interest, and that we are more empathic with or towards those who are close to us, whom we live with, or with whom we are intimately associated in other ways than we are to strangers or people we do not know personally, and "this difference can (therefore) mean that we prefer to help the former, even if we are in a position to do somewhat more good for the latter" (Slote 2010, 131). This can justify "Dr. Kate" being more empathetic towards her sick cousin in room 301 than to the victim of a motor vehicle accident in room 805, whom she has never met (and the actions that might ensue). To the students of Dr. Kate, this might not be a good educational opportunity either. Slote argues that empathy, or caring, is "the basis of moral right or wrong" (2013, 22). It consists of mirroring the feelings of another person, of an emotional identification with the predicaments and suffering of the other, neurologically activated through the mirror neuron mechanism that forms the basis for altruistic motivation and action. Yet medical practice is full of instances where physicians do not have empathy "aroused in themselves" because they are caring for unconscious patients or those in a persistent vegetative state. In addition, there are times when morality requires the physician to weaken her empathic connection and rely on reason and practical wisdom in order to be able to care for her patient. So while Slote's moral sentimentalism can be used in teaching students of medicine to be more empathetic towards their patients, and while his assertion that moral action has its origin in family and peers is plausible and defensible, these do not help us in graduating the virtuous physician who might matriculate into medical school with character flaws. Other virtue ethicists, such as Philippa Foot, Alasdair MacIntyre, and Rosalind Hursthouse similarily have their own contemporary philosophies, none of which provide a framework to guide us in our project aiming at the moral education of the future physician. Foot expounded a naturalistic theory of ethics whereby goodness is seen as the natural flourishing of humans, and virtues must engage the will, depend on human nature, and be *corrective* in that they exist to fight a temptation or a defect in motivation. She compares humans to planks of wood that naturally change form and require constant efforts to keep them straight. Virtues do the same for human character. However, she does not tell us *how* this "strengthening" takes place. Consider Drs. Helen and Kate, who work at the same teaching hospital.

Each has the opportunity to charge patients without examining them by simply asking students to have patients sign the consultation form. The idea never occurs to Dr. Helen and, one can argue, she is naturally virtuous. However, Dr. Kate, who has a mortgage to pay, is often lured by the temptation of making extra money but overcomes this temptation. The virtue of Dr. Kate lies in her overcoming temptation. But, in Aristotle's framework, she is a *continent* person and lacks internal harmony. If, as Foot maintains (Foot, 1978, 320), virtue is a "corrective" disposition, then Dr. Kate is not fully disposed to be honest and thus cannot be virtuous in Aristotle's terms since the virtuous person wants to do what is right and takes pleasure in it. In "Virtues and Vices," she asks *whether the benefit of the virtues go to the person with the virtue or to the people who are affected by that person*, and argues that with some virtues, like courage, temperance, and wisdom, the answer is apparent, as they benefit both the person who has these dispositions and others as well. With justice and charity, the answer is not as clear. It seems as if the charitable person benefits the other more than himself and "may seem to be deleterious to their possessor." It might even be that the charitable person loses in the performance of the virtue. For neophyte students—with their immaturity and inexperience, human nature being what it is, and with the current conditions of life—to sense that practicing such virtues is deleterious is damaging to the nurturing of the virtues. Foot also argues that a person's moral dispositions are judged by his intentions, which, in the educational project we are aiming at, sounds a little bit elusive. Would we really want students of medicine to judge (and learn from) the behavior of a physician based on her "intentions"? And how sound or right is that?

MacIntyre, on the other hand, argues that virtues are acquired qualities that allow us to achieve goods internal to practices and are developed through shared practices. We learn by doing and by pondering our behavior jointly with others through a "practice."[6] Reflecting on the practice is an essential part of moral development. A person, he tell us, is a "story-telling animal" (MacIntyre 1984, 216) and it is important to know what stories one finds oneself in. This "narrative quest" (1984, 218) allows for an education of character and self-knowledge. After looking at a

---

6. A practice is "any coherent and complex form of socially established cooperative human activity through which goods internal to that form of activity are realized in the course of trying to achieve those standards of excellence which are appropriate to and partially definitive of that form of activity, with the result that human powers to achieve excellence, and human conceptions of the ends and goods involved, are systematically extended" (1984, 187). Examples are chess, painting, music, farming and medicine, among others. A practice is intentional, and goods internal to that activity are basically realized. He then continues: "A virtue is an acquired human quality the possession and exercise of which tends to enable us to achieve those goods which are internal to practices and the lack of which effectively prevents us from achieving any such goods" (p. 191). With medicine as a "practice," its good is completed whenever a number of patients are cared for on a daily basis (when the ends of medicine are met). Yet, the success of this practice does not depend on it alone, as medicine is not an edifice that stands on its own—universities, research institutes, drug companies, insurance companies, governments, and other stakeholders have roles to play.

number of historical accounts of virtue, he concludes that the prevailing differences are the result of dissimilar practices which engender different conceptions of virtues. Virtues—the most important ones, he now says, are justice, honesty, and courage—require explanation of social and moral features in order to be understood and are dependent on the context of the society in which they are exercised. For example, Homeric virtues are understood by looking at their social roles in ancient Greek society. How stable are such virtues and to what extent can we count on them to build the character of a physician who will *do the right thing even when no one is looking*? Consider a physician who has been practicing in the Kingdom of Saudi Arabia for twenty years; MacIntyre's virtue theory entails that she will have to change her virtues when she starts practicing in the US. This has unpleasant repercussions on the character and stable dispositions that we are trying to build, and MacIntyre does not deal with such problems. His theory on virtue rests on the excellence involved in any established practice (medicine being one) and the importance of living a coherent narrative given one's individual culture and obligations. Virtues help to "sustain the households and communities" together and will also increase "self-knowledge . . . and knowledge of the good" (1984, 219). This would imply that a physician aiding a woman to abort a fetus with birth defects is virtuous based on the argument that she is keeping the community together because the woman's husband has threatened to divorce her if she keeps the child. Again, MacIntyre does not deal with such concerns. According to him, we live "after virtue" because of modern-day individualism, as the self has no tradition to learn the virtues from.

In his "How to Seem Virtuous Without Actually Being So" (1999), MacIntyre contends that society comprises:

> *a number of rival and incompatible accounts of the virtues . . . [T]here can be no rationally defensible shared programme for moral education for our society as such, but only a number of rival and conflicting programmes, each from the standpoint of one specific contending view (1999, 118).*

This is so precisely because a conception of the human *telos* is lacking in a pluralistic society marked by "counterfeit rhetoric." Education into virtues "has to begin by discovering some way of transforming the motivations of those who are to be so educated" (1999, 123), and educators face the problem of being unable to make students value the virtues as such or to create in them the motivation to be genuinely virtuous. Students will consider particular situations but will fail to understand what it is about the actions that make them "genuine examples of some particular virtue"

(1999, 123). He concludes that "what the morality of the virtues articulated in and defended by the moral rhetoric of our political culture provides is, it turns out, not an education in the virtues, but rather, an education in how to seem virtuous without actually being so" (1999, 131), which is not what we want for our future physicians. Waiting for a new "St. Benedict" cannot be the solution; so while MacIntyre's theory has many merits, it does not offer a framework that will allow us to construct a plan to graduate the physician who will do the right thing even if no one is looking. What about Hursthouse?

Like Aristotle, Hursthouse maintains that when persons act virtuously, they act in accordance with the characteristics of their nature as human beings, and this will lead to *eudaimonia*. According to her, it is a strength of virtue ethics that it does not resolve all moral dilemmas since this is actually a correct portrayal of moral life: "Here we come to an interesting defense of the v-rules, often criticized as being too difficult to apply for the agent who lacks moral wisdom.[7] The defense relies on an (insufficiently acknowledged) insight of Aristotle's—namely that moral knowledge, unlike mathematical knowledge, cannot be acquired merely by attending lectures and is not characteristically to be found in people too young to have much experience of life" (1996, 650). While she refers to the acquisition of moral knowledge, Hursthouse does not explicitly devote any attention to moral education and we are not told what to do with the young who do not have much experience with life (like the neophyte student of medicine having a set of v-rules whose guidance seems to raise conflicts). Still, without using the actual term, she has alluded to role models in her "Virtue Theory and Abortion" (2011), warning against taking literally the maxim *do what the virtuous agent would do in the circumstances*: "[V]irtue theory is not limited to considering '[w]ould Socrates have had an abortion if he were a raped, pregnant fifteen-year-old?'" (2011, 244). Thus, although Hursthouse does not counter Aristotle's moral education, notions of habituation, and role models, she does not offer her own full theory (at least in print).

Accordingly, while Slote, Foot, MacIntyre, and Hursthouse have clearly a lot to offer, none of them offers a theory that allows us to graduate the physician who will *do the right thing even when no one is looking*. Aristotle's theory, with its emphasis on rationality, character development through habituation, the role of *phronesis* in deliberation, *akrasia* and its effects, and the importance of virtues in leading a happy

---

7. V-rules are virtue rules that dictate: "Do what is honest/charitable; do not do what is dishonest/uncharitable" (Hursthouse 1999).

and harmonious life, seems to me to be a good model to support what I want to argue.

All in all, Aristotle offers a good framework. I do not rely on all of Aristotle's ethics; in fact, and most importantly, this book is not on virtue ethics per se; rather it is an attempt to deal with the problem of a corrupt medical profession and how to remedy the situation by educating the good medical student who will be brought up to do what is right. Hence in what follows, I will try to show how Aristotle's virtue ethics has in it the seeds of a good and sustainable structure for the making of the good physician. This may be only one of several ways of solving this problem.

Aristotle's virtue ethics is certainly relevant to the medical profession. Linking moral virtues with the kind of person the physician ought to be and with the excellence of her work has practical implications for the making of the "good physician." Consequently, one can argue that admissions criteria have a bearing on the sort of student who enters medical school to begin with since moral fiber has a bearing on the kind of physician he will be in the future.[8] In other words, since character is partly formed by family, friends, close associates, school, neighborhood, church, and other formative influences, then not just anyone should be admitted into medical school; a sort of sifting—a screening process—should take place prior to admission. Medical College Admission Test (MCAT) scores, however important, should not constitute the sole parameter to judge by, nor should medical interviews that cannot assess the character of the applicant. It is implied by Aristotle's approach that students who enter medical school with no knowledge can be taught it, but if they enter medical school with an appalling character—for example, a psychopath like the notorious case of Dr. Swango—they cannot be taught good character. The likelihood of success in remedying flaws of character during education would depend on several factors, the three most important being:

1) The extent to which the individual's character has been formed. Several studies have shown that the character of a student has not been totally fixed by the time he enters the late teens and early twenties and that some changes remain to take place (Branch 2000; Feudtner et al. 1994). Students must have a propensity for identifying virtuous behavior, be motivated to become virtuous, and be willing to subjugate their emotions and desires to the rule of reason. This does not mean that they will have to suppress their emotions, for indeed these are important and must be experienced in a proper way, for character formation involves developing

---

8. More will be said about the importance of admissions criteria and their relationship to the character of the applicant to medical schools in chapter four.

certain interests, refining some desires, and accepting some emotions. According to Aristotle, virtuous people take pleasure in what they do (1947, 526).

2) The competence, determination, and resourcefulness of the educator. The educator and role model has to demonstrate wide knowledge and expertise as well as *phronesis*. She should be armed with moral courage and have a commitment to uphold and act upon her ethical beliefs. Thus, the gap between what is said and what is done is bridged, and the educator must protect at-risk ethical values. She should be a person determined to make a difference.

3) The extent to which education takes place in a supportive and sustaining environment (with appropriate role models and under credible sanctions). The educator or role model will not thrive or exert the necessary influence on medical students unless she is working within a supportive environment, otherwise opposing forces will obstruct her efforts to make a difference.

Here two important issues arise: (1) Admissions criteria should give preference to candidates of high moral character,[9] and (2) once accepted into medical school, students cannot be guaranteed that they will graduate; rather, they should be reminded that they will graduate *if and only if* they meet the curriculum requirements. In other words, if they falter in morals, they should be asked to leave.[10] To my knowledge, no medical school to date attempts to do this. Given current practice in medical schools, how can we work on shaping the character of the students who are already there? Returning to the ends of medicine, as discussed in chapter one, we realize that the student of medicine has to possess a number of virtues that will ensure he will not fall prey either to personal interest or to the "sins of modern medicine." According to Pellegrino, these sins are many and include but are not limited to: "overspecialization; technicism; overprofessionalization; insensitivity to personal and sociocultural values; too narrow a construal of the doctor's role; too much "curing" rather than "caring"; not enough emphasis on prevention, patient participation, and patient education; too much science, not enough liberal arts; not enough behavioral science; too much economic incentive; a "trade school" mentality; insensitivity to the poor and socially disadvantaged; overmedicalization of everyday life; inhumane treatment of medical students; overworked house staff; and deficiencies in verbal and nonverbal communication" (1979, 9–10). Medicine is becoming morally bankrupt, with physicians turning into entrepreneurs because they feel that they have to fulfill the demands of the

---

9. Some schools have started using a Defining Issues Test (DIT), but even this and similar tests fail to truly assess the ethical sensitivity of the student.

10. More will be said about these issues in chapter four.

"market." It is also argued that the pluralism that characterizes modern society makes defending the acquisition of a unique set of virtues difficult. Hence, there is a need for what I call "core traits" or "core virtues." We are not looking for a *unique* set of virtues. Rather, we are attempting to find "*core* virtues" that play the role of universals within medicine. Yet, one can justifiably wonder, if these *core virtues* were to be internalized, what guarantee would we have that virtuous physicians would not be lured by external forces, and that the virtues would not be lost? Would these be virtues in the first place or simply *accidental traits*? As was mentioned previously, the Aesculapian myth by the poet Pindar depicts the god of medicine driven away from the Aristotelian virtue of moderation and fallen prey to vice. Thus, we read about the tragedy of Aesculapius:

> *Even the lore of leechcraft is enthralled by the love of gain; even he was seduced by a splendid fee of gold displayed upon the palm to bring back from death one who was already its lawful prey. Therefore the son of Cronus with his hands hurled his shaft through both of them, and swiftly reft the breath from out their breasts, for they were stricken with sudden doom by the gleaming thunderbolt (Pindar 1924, 191).*

To this one might add that if the *telos* of the physician-patient relationship, as presented in the ends of medicine, is ultimately healing and helping to relieve suffering, then core virtues play an important role in the fulfillment of these ends. They offer a guarantee that the student of medicine, the future physician, will not falter even when no one is looking. As they are internalized and become second nature, the physician will not be able to act except based on these virtues. It is this that will make her fulfill her function as a physician and lead a harmonious happy life with her profession. The good virtuous physician will be one who demonstrates the core character traits that most successfully realize the ends of medicine. Some of these virtues, as presented by Pellegrino and Thomasma, are fidelity to trust, compassion, *phronesis*, justice, fortitude, temperance, integrity and self-effacement (1993).[11]

So how do students of medicine learn these excellences or core virtues? It is here that Aristotle's theory of virtue as habituation (along with the crowning characteristic of *phronesis*) comes in. Medical students need to be habituated to do the right thing, and habit will make doing the right thing second nature. With time, they will develop the

---

11. Francis Walker (2005) suggests the cultivation of the additional virtues of tact, good humor, self-awareness, simplicity, reverence, and courage.

capacity to deliberate over complex situations and reach appropriate conclusions. In *phronesis*, the intellectual and the moral virtues are united and the moral agent is capable of prioritizing the virtues and of making the right decision when faced with situations that offer complex moral conundrums. Medical students then will be able to make the right clinical decisions that earlier on seemed too difficult to make. Virtuous physicians will be safeguarded from the possible metamorphosis that might mean that another physician falls prey to the sins of medicine. In that sense, core virtues function like safety valves against the sins of modern medicine. Notwithstanding, this presupposes that medical students who are already in medical school have some predisposition to becoming good physicians. According to Aristotle, we do not acquire a virtue that is contrary to nature. For Aristotle, humans do not have an innate character imbedded in their nature that makes them the kind of persons they are and hence not amenable to change. Rather, at birth, persons possess a potentiality out of which a set of qualities—character—develops. The mere fact that a character changes proves this. As Aristotle says, a "stone which by nature moves downwards cannot be habituated to move upwards" (1947, 331). The stone totally lacks the potential of learning how to fly. This task, which is not only challenging, but also impossible, is doomed to failure. No teacher or trainer can be so effective. If character were innate, it would not be open to change, just like the stone, but it is not. People can be educated; they can be brought up to become virtuous adults, but not all people nor students of medicine will grow up to become virtuous individuals and virtuous physicians. Consider the case of the acorn: a proper environment that provides the necessary conditions is required in order for its potential to be realized, for the acorn to become an oak tree. Yet, one cannot but wonder about the character of the student of medicine who enters medical school and is resistant to change. The fact remains that there are persons who should not be in medical school at all, who are characterologically flawed and who, in a sense, can never be corrected, an issue that will be dealt with in chapter four. There are also unsuccessful experiments of students who were initially admitted to medical school as "works in progress," but who nonetheless did not develop the hoped-for virtues. Such students should not be permitted to graduate and to deal with the lives and health of vulnerable patients. These are not a majority, but they should not be ignored, and appropriate action should be taken regarding them. Would one tolerate a medical student who ridicules the narratives of patients, who thinks character is irrelevant and sincerely believes that ethics has no place in medicine, which he views as solely a scientific endeavor devoid of moral scruples? A medical student who enters medical school with an unsuitable character, with no desire to change, and who only sees medicine as a gateway to prestige and power might be an experiment doomed to fail, and, perhaps like Aristotle's Alexander, a tragic hero. Aristotle's greatest pupil and his utmost failure, Alexander, was a vigorous personality who unified what had previously been scattered city-states, but in so doing also caused the demise of democracy. He had several flaws to his personality, yet, perhaps Alexander's main tragic flaw was what Aristotle calls "weakness of will" (*akrasia*). Aristotle defines an *akratic* agent as one who "knowing that what he does is bad, does it as a result of passions" (1947, 443). He thought of *akrasia* as lack of self-control and that the persons who exhibit a lack of self-control (*akrates*) would not possess practical wisdom. An *akratic* student (who knows what he ought to do but fails to do it because of his unruly feelings) will be torn by conflict, as his rational and emotional faculties will not speak the same language. This is precisely why, says Aristotle, such persons are unhappy while virtuous persons are happy and at peace with themselves. One question that might arise in connection to *akrasia* is the following: is it possible for a physician knowingly not to do what she thinks is best for the patient? One might answer this by saying that, in principle, this is not possible. Yet, practically, a physician with a flawed character can be lured to do that which she knows is not best for a particular patient. Take the example of patient A, suffering from an organ failure and in need of an immediate organ transplant. Security at the hospital is tight, and the physician of that particular patient happens to have another patient B who is terminally ill and will die in a few days anyway. Patient B is a perfect match for patient A. The physician is told by the family of patient A that should he secure the organ and should the transplant be successful he will be awarded a generous amount of money. Lured by the prospect of economic gain, and convincing herself that patient B will die anyway in a few days, she hastens the death of patient B, removes the organ, and gives it to patient A. This would not have happened had the doctor internalized the core virtues. A virtuous physician does not find it difficult to do the right thing, indeed not to do so is against her nature. She will not simply have virtues; she will *become* her virtues. For Aristotle, the virtues entice the person to do his work well and make him a good person: "[t]herefore it is true in every case, the virtue of man also will be the state of character which makes a man good and which makes him do his own work well" (1947, 338). As such, the virtuous physician will not be metamorphosed under any circumstances, but will stand firm even when no one is looking, even if security is not tight and she can get away with it. Notwithstanding, this is not to say that virtue ethics alone will suffice in guiding the conduct of the future physician. Rules and duties will also play an important role in that they offer some guidance to the neophyte student who is still building his character. In addition, even when fully formed in terms of character, the physician cannot act regardless of the rules and duties set by the organization, society, and profession in which she is practicing. These rules and duties are moral as well as institutional and professional in nature. Being part of an institution and profession entails agreeing to work within certain moral parameters set by the institution and profession. Even if this agreement does not reach the status of an enforceable contract, there is an obligation to do the things that are agreed upon, especially when patients, members of the healthcare team, and others involved are relying on them to do so, the assumption being that these rules and duties are such that they do not violate general moral decorum. The physician will have to exercise prudence but still regard and respect the rules and duties that are present and endorsed for a reason. Here one can recall the moral absolutes presented by Pellegrino and how such absolutes can hamper good doctoring instead of promoting it. If neophyte physicians were to blindly bow to moral absolutes, irrespective of the context and the status quo, their prudential thinking would be obstructed in that they would not have the chance to practice and develop their *phronesis* under the guidance of mentors and they would not be able to make decisions that would be in the best interest of *this* patient at *this* moment, the point being that, alone, rules and duties will not make a good physician who will do the right thing even if no one is looking.[12] As Pellegrino and Thomasma state, "even if there might be agreement on a definition of the good, there is a certain circularity in the logic of virtue ethics. The morally good act is one done by the virtuous person; the virtuous person is one who performs morally good acts. This circular reasoning is tolerable when some common notion of the good is accepted by all. When there is no such common notion, the logical consistency of the connections between character and morally good acts is no longer sustainable" (1993, 18). Thus, a justification for acts needs to be sought outside the virtues, and here comes the role of principles or rules as action guides *in addition* to virtues. Virtues remain the central element, for it is precisely the agent himself who will choose what principles or rules to follow. Here, one inevitable question arises: Why virtue ethics? The answer to this question lies in the fact that the view of moral education that is being taken in this book is that one has to be a certain kind of being in order to do the right thing. One of the main goals of this book is to argue that character needs to be regarded as one of the aims of the education of physicians (in addition to the skills and science that they need to earn an MD degree). These traits of

---

12. Add to this the possibility that a physician might be tempted to ignore the rules in favor of self-interest and personal gain if she is sure that no one will know about her infraction, as with the shepherd's use of the ring of Gyges, referred to earlier. The same can be said about ignoring one's duties if this can go unnoticed.

character are scalar qualities (that one can have more or less of), characterized in aretaic terms, and they are virtues. In addition to focusing on the moral formation of the person *qua* person, virtue ethics also focuses on the moral formation of the person as part of a social fabric. Alasdair McIntyre spoke of the cooperation of people for the attainment of goods that are internal to those of the practice they belong to. Thus, the virtues are the qualities of the physician both as a person and a professional, and this is what we aim at bringing about. As mentioned earlier, while rules might matter, they alone do not offer much that can be relied on because it is a matter of what kind of person one actually is that makes the difference.[13] At the end of the day, rules (institutional or legal or even moral, if one is of a weak moral fiber) can be broken (misused or abused) if no one is looking because—human nature being what it is, the economic situation being what it is, life's burdens being what they are—students of medicine and physicians are and will be influenced by many circumstances. Unless they are specific kinds of persons whose character will guarantee that they will be morally equipped to resist temptation no matter what, nothing will guarantee their obedience to the rules or their doing the right thing. One has to be realistic. In contrast to Rousseau, the assumption here, again, is that virtues are not natural, and human beings are not born good or just. Yet, in contrast to Hobbes, they are not born evil either: "Neither by nature, then, nor contrary to nature do the virtues arise in us; rather we are adapted by nature to receive them and are made perfect by habit" (Aristotle 1947, 331). One can argue that some internalizing or truly believing in principles might have the same motivational effect as coming to acquire a virtue. The answer to this is that principles can, at best, offer proper moral guidance to a virtuous moral agent. What guarantees that the principles one adopts are the morally correct ones? Is it morally right for a physician to adopt a principle stating that the "end justifies the means" when the end for her is to make more money? It is indeed not right to appeal to the principle that "the end justifies the means" when the end is a bad one. Yet, the question arises whether a morally good end can be justifiably realized via bad means. This is when matters get a little difficult. For example, it is debatable whether a lie told in the pursuit of another virtue (*ceteris paribus,* not telling a patient he suffers from a serious disease out of compassion because you know the patient well and have reason to believe that he will harm himself) is right or wrong. It remains the case that it is nearly impossible to get theoretical exactness on practical matters. The virtuous physician will have to ponder the case at hand and be aware of the particulars that construct the case

---

13. It is not about action, but about character. Once character is guaranteed, actions will naturally come about.

(which unfortunately rarely happens in contemporary medicine where patients are most of the time treated as "diseases" or "cases" regardless of their narratives and situations). The physician must ensure that she recognizes the facts, sees and understands what is morally relevant, and makes decisions that are sensitive to the demands of each particular case. Lying to a patient might not be virtuous in *all* circumstances, but with this particular patient, this particular case, and at this particular time, it is the virtuous thing to do. The virtues are exhibited in behavior, and when facing an apparent conflict between virtues (a compassionate lie), virtue ethics asks us to imagine how a virtuous person would act in this situation, then make that person's virtues our own and, since moral judgments are often difficult and "the decision rests with perception" (1947, 347), one must rely on personal judgment to decide what is right. Some virtues are needed as a starting point.

Principles tend to be rigid, and what is needed for a physician is flexibility in moral deliberations. Thus, moral character is acquired through education, and humans (in this case, students of medicine) can be educated to become virtuous and to develop the appropriate emotional response relevant to the situation. The strength of virtue ethics is that it delineates that there are no absolute rules in ethics, but that ethics is a matter of practical wisdom which involves a mixture of understanding and experience; involves the ability to read individual situations aptly; draws on previous experiences; and allows the person to constantly improve his understanding in the light of each individual situation that he faces. That person "sees" what should be done on "each" occasion. He has developed an internal compass, so to speak. Theories that give rules are at best unrealistic for a very simple reason: there can be no such thing as a magic recipe for right action since situations vary and no two instances are exactly the same. For example, absolute deontology is inattentive to situations and state of affairs: lying cannot be wrong in all circumstances, and sticking to absolutes might be problematic, particularly in the practice of medicine. For example, one's duty to respect autonomy (e.g., abiding by the wishes of an HIV patient not to tell his spouse about his condition) might be outweighed in certain situations by our duty to help or save others (the spouse getting infected). One might argue that some of the strengths found in virtue ethics are found in other moral frameworks, such as that of W. D. Ross and moral particularism. Ross was equally sensitive to context. According to him, the consequences of an action (lying) may sometimes make lying the right thing to do. He differentiates between "prima facie duties" and "duties proper." Prima facie duties are not absolute but must be considered alongside other duties. Yet, insofar as prima facie duties conflict, one must decide on the basis of contextual details which of these duties is most pressing. The action that is judged to be, all things considered, the right thing to do is the duty proper, and we know what our duty is by "intuition." However, we intuit general obligations and not what is right in a particular situation, as reasoning is needed. "Principlism" has gained almost worldwide acceptance, and acknowledgment and is being taught in almost all medical schools as a guideline to dealing with cases laden with ethical controversy. Yet, while one might agree on the main principles presented by Beauchamp and Childress (1994), one might dispute the range of their application. In the case of an unmarried pregnant woman who is on drugs and who requests an abortion because she cannot raise her child, the question would be *to whom do we owe the duty of beneficence, to her or to the fetus*? Another example would be the case of conflicting duties. When faced with moral dilemmas and we have a conflict between duties of equal importance, we are morally obligated to disregard one duty. There are no magic recipes, and such scenarios are more frequent today as moral life is getting more and more complicated and characterized by too many particulars. Another example would be patient-centered deontological theories where rights matter more than duties. Hence, a physician must not allow herself to be used for moral good against her will. Should she be the only emergency department physician present when a serial rapist is rushed in, no virtue talk can convince her to save the life of the patient then turn him in to the authorities *if* she does not want to. The point, at least in this situation, is that the consequences of the action are significant enough to be taken into consideration. Not doing so will imply, at the least, that the physician has betrayed the internal ends of medicine.

Indeed, for our purposes and project, Aristotle's virtue ethics has an edge over other theories in that it primarily recognizes the facts that, as human beings, we have a capacity to reason, influenced by our emotions, and that ethical perception consists of cognitive processes and emotional registration. Thus, when faced with a patient's case, the physician will perceive the situation, judge what is right, and want to act in the right way because that course of action is second nature to her. In the long run, without the internationalization of virtues, straight obedience to rules becomes sterile. With virtue ethics, the physician unravels the particulars of the case, uses moral imagination, appreciates the importance of emotion as well as reason, and uses practical wisdom that is the product of a learning process. Henceforth, virtue ethics offers an inclusive framework.

Consider the case of 45-year-old Mrs. Jones, who was five months pregnant when she was rushed to the emergency department, suffering from what appeared to be a stroke. The attending physician and her team deduced that serious medical problems with the fetus were causing her illness and suggested terminating the pregnancy to save her life. Mrs. Jones refused, and her decision was backed by the chair of the division, Dr. Catharine, who looked at the particulars of the case: Mrs. Jones's pregnancy was a result of a third IVF trial; she had lost her husband and could not afford, emotionally, to lose the child. Mrs. Jones and Dr. Catharine fought for her fetus, and both survived. Understanding the context necessitates a thorough mapping of the case in a way that allows one to see the salient features. General rules and guidelines might be handy, but it is crucial to reflect on the situation and to use moral imagination, reasoning, emotion, and practical wisdom. It is also important to note that, since our project is one concerned with forming a certain kind of physician, character building is essential; we do not want a physician to visit a terminally-ill patient whose treatment is deemed futile because it is her *duty*, but because it is the *compassionate* thing to do, and she embodies the virtue of compassion (mean and all). The practice of medicine places the medical student in situations that are morally different and multifaceted. Students need to grasp the moral issues intrinsic in these situations or else they will only be attuned to the science of the case, and the internal ends of medicine will not be met. Flexibility in evaluating the case at hand by considering what a virtuous agent would do in this situation allows new and diverse solutions to cases that cannot be solved by mere obedience to rules and principles. Cases like that of Mrs. Jones are emotionally laden, but as Aristotle would have it, emotion is not only a manner of reacting; it is also a manner of perceiving, of being involved, and then reacting in a particular situation. Thus, to act rightly involves acting rightly in affect; it is learning to feel the right emotions in the right situations.

Virtue ethics comes on the scene as a more opportune moral theory. It is timely because individuals are being tempted to do the wrong thing when no one is watching, when they can get away with it, particularly with some personal gain or with no loss to themselves. Not all thinkers agree with this. For example, Robert Louden (1984, 227–236) argues that, at best, virtue ethics has an auxiliary role to play and that the chief role is actually played by an ethics of rules. The main critique of virtue ethics is that it does not offer sufficient guidance to people, particularly when facing different and new situations, an idea discussed by Hursthouse (1995, 56–75).[14] While it is true that virtue ethics will not provide either the neophyte

---

14. Some critique it as being culturally relative because different cultures have different values. But this problem of

or the veteran physician with a modus operandi for determining what the right action is, this is in fact one of the virtues of virtue ethics because offering such algorithms, to use Onora O'Neill's term, seems unrealistic since the right action really cannot be codified within a formula or an algorithm, as there are always many surrounding variables (O'Neill 1987, 55–69). The main strength of the virtue ethics approach in contrast to utilitarian and the deontological ones, for example,[15] is that it constantly recognizes that life is full of tension, that there is a plurality of goods (at times conflicting goods), and that however hard a person tries, she cannot have all the goods all the time.[16] Henceforth, the fact that virtue ethics does not help us discover the right thing to do might actually be viewed as its strength, for ethical questions are a function of the situation and ought to be continually subject to re-examination. Aristotle himself gives the analogy of the steersman: the ethicist (and for our purposes, the good physician) is like a steersman trying to take a boat through a hazardous stretch. He has his eyes on a plethora of things: the state of the water, the indication of the compass, the force of the wind, light conditions, and other factors. It is the capacity to appreciate the complexity of the situation and to make a good decision that makes him a wise steersman. Simple adherence to rules and principles will not always do the trick since, as was previously argued, there can be no such thing as a magic recipe for right action in view of the fact that, for a practicing physician dealing with patients, no two patients or cases are exactly the same, and even a considered application of rules or principles will not always suffice, even when supplemented with additional nuances and refinements for dealing with conflicting principles.[17] This is so because of the nature of medicine and the cases one is faced with. Each patient is unique, with particular needs and values. Michael Stocker (1976), who argued that utilitarianism and deontology concentrate on rules, obligations, and principles instead of persons, criticized these theories, noting that they make harmony between reason and motive almost impossible, which leads to a "malady of the spirit," causing the agent to develop a schism between his actions and motivations (1976, 454), and are thus defective. Virtue ethics, by focusing on the character and disposition of the person, does not suffer from this deficiency. Rules, while useful, are not enough, and Aristotle tells us that ethics is not a matter

relativity is not peculiar to virtue ethics since cultural disparity in character traits is not greater than the one we see in rules of behavior (thus deontology is not immune), and one can also argue that different cultures have different notions about what makes up for happiness or welfare.

15. After all, the application of such principles or rules requires what Aristotle called practical wisdom.

16. An example discussed earlier is principlism and the controversy around the scope of the application of the main principles this theory offers.

17. As Hursthouse puts it, "[w]hy should it be a condition of adequacy on a moral theory that it should provide an algorithm for life?" She continues, saying that: "[r]ather than criticizing a secular theory for failing to come up with rules that settle difficult cases, we might say that it is entirely to its credit that it does not do so" (1995, 61).

of generalization, that we must "not look for precision in all things alike, but in each class of things such precision as accords with the subject matter, and so much as is appropriate to the inquiry" (1947, 319). Cases will have to be dealt with "in the right times, with reference to the right objects, towards the right people, with the right motive, and in the right way, is what is both intermediate and best, and this is characteristic of virtue" (1947, 340). Learning to live a good life is a kind of extensive moral apprenticeship. At the beginning, one sometimes acts correctly yet perhaps without deep sincerity, but as time passes by, and as one learns, one becomes a person of integrity: one's actions, thoughts, and feelings become synchronized.[18] All this requires experience and practical wisdom, but eventually this person can be relied on to do the right thing in all circumstances. Yet, is virtue ethics alone enough? It might be necessary, but it is not sufficient particularly to the neophyte who has not yet acquired enough experience or practical wisdom. And since a good deal of medical ethics necessarily ought to be about the patient and based on *duties* owed directly to other human beings, virtue ethics is more or less directed towards the self and the cultivation of core virtues. Add to that the fact that human beings are fallible, and as virtuous as a character can be and as prudent as a person can be, this does not make her immune from errors in judgment. Thus, the language of duty and obligation *in addition to* that of virtues comes in handy. Virtue ethics suggests that duties will be respected somewhat effortlessly and that whenever duties conflict, the right decision will be made by the *phronimos* the student of medicine has now become. Hence, if one is to build character as proposed above, then one has to begin by teaching the virtues. The assumption is, of course, that one has identified what the right virtues are and verified that these virtues can be translated into attitudes; it is one thing to appreciate cleanliness and another thing not to litter. So at this point, two important questions arise. Can virtue be taught? And if yes, how?

2.4. Can We Teach Virtue?

In Plato's *Meno*, the title character asks Socrates a question left unanswered: "Can you tell me, Socrates, whether virtue is acquired by teaching or practice, or if by neither teaching nor practice, whether it comes to us by nature or some other way?" (Plato 2013, 70). Aristotle answers this question: Intellectual virtue can be learned (and improved) as a result of methodical instruction whereas moral virtue is a matter of habituation and practice, the best practice being the imitation of a good

---

18. The importance of role models will be discussed later in this chapter and in chapter three.

role model.[19] Thus, for Aristotle, virtue can be taught; while it is not natural, it is not opposed to nature either. Nevertheless, Aristotle was aware that it takes a long period of time for a moral character to develop since human beings are born with numerous tendencies and a person's ability to regulate his desires is not as easy as one might think. Wayne Shelton, arguing for the importance of teaching virtues to medical students and acknowledging the fact that modern-day society is a pluralistic one, presenting a need to respect the individual in the student, sees in Aristotle's virtue ethics "guidance for medical educators" (1999, 672), and he proposes the use of Aristotle's framework of virtue as a yardstick for training new physicians (1999, 672). Delese Wear and Joseph Zarconi (2008) conjecture that compassion and other virtues can indeed be taught to medical students, and they argue that once curriculum time is over, medical students rely on role models to learn the virtues. Still, even if we grant that virtue can be taught, the issue of whether it will or should be taught remains a matter of much controversy. We find a similar debate in Plato's *Republic*: according to Glaucon, we do what is right only under pressure, while Thrasymachus argued that goodness is a charade, and what matters is having a good reputation. Many modern physicians adhere to Thrasymachus's vision, and many students of medicine are *akratic*.[20] It is precisely these physicians who are causing damage to the profession of medicine. Regardless of Aristotle's own vision of the development of virtue, it remains a fact that if virtue is to be taught, there need to be at least two mechanisms to teach it: (1) a role model (as Aristotle himself suggested), and (2) an organizational structure and culture that will allow the flourishing of such virtues.

2.4.1. Role Models

A role model can be defined as someone who "teaches primarily by example and helps to shape professional identity and commitment through promoting observation and comparison. Unlike mentors, role models may have only brief contact with physicians in training and do not so much deliberately mold students as inspire by their own conduct" (Reuler and Nardone, 1994, 335). As stated by Scott Wright and Joseph Carrese, "physician role models affect the attitudes, behaviors and ethics of medical learners and foster professional values in trainees. They also influence

---

19. Intellectual virtue meaning "science, art, practical wisdom, intuitive wisdom, theoretical wisdom." Plato's cardinal virtues are wisdom, justice, fortitude, and temperance. In this book, when reference is made to virtue, it is primarily moral virtue that is intended.

20. Defined by the Oxford English Dictionary as "Exhibiting or characterized by lack of restraint or weakness of will. Also: characterized by the tendency to act against one's better judgement."

the career choices of medical students" (2002, 638). Aristotle's virtue ethics relies significantly on the effects that role models have on human beings. One of the main tenets of Aristotelian philosophy is that people learn by emulating moral exemplars. Since people learn by practice, the best practice is to imitate role models. It is in that sense that through a process of continuous imitation of the virtuous physician, the student becomes habitually virtuous himself. Henceforth, the virtuous physician will model good behavior and will also be able to explain to the neophyte physician the reasons for behaving the way she does. It may appear from this that it is action, rather than character, that is the primary means of instilling desirable character traits in others. However, this is not what is intended here. Character is fundamental, and with the established veteran physician, actions emanate from a firm character. The practice of medicine requires the exercise of reasoning and judgment in clinical as well as ethical capacities, and *phronesis* cannot be taught. It is basically practical understanding in situ that involves a lot of deliberation on the part of the *phronimos*. It is, after all, "the work of the man of practical wisdom, to deliberate well" (1947, 431). Thus, good character cannot be attained outside the experience in which it plays a role. Being a role model and having chosen to behave the way she does, based on knowledge, experience, and *phronesis*, the physician is able to explain and willing to clarify the reasons for her choices to students so as to ensure that they understand the reasons for her behavior. This will present opportunities for discussion and reflection, and hence will improve learning. Students will have a chance to develop their own *phronesis* with time and under the guidance of a dedicated role model. Thus, ends are set by character, and *phronesis* allows us to pursue those ends: "choice will not be right without practical wisdom any more than without virtue; for the one determines the end and the other makes us do the things that lead to the end" (1947, 442).

Students can easily identify role models: they sense enthusiasm, passion, and honesty, which is evidently contagious. Wright examined what medical residents look for in their role models. With 230 questionnaires distributed at McGill University and a response rate of 85%, he found that "aggregate responses of all residents showed that clinical skills, personality, and teaching ability were ranked as the top three factors by over 90%" of respondents (1996, 291), and concluded that "attending physicians who are excellent role models need to be identified at all institutions so that they can be selected to spend more time with medical students and residents" (1996, 292). Teaching psychosocial skills was also viewed by students as great faculty role modeling (Wright et al., 1998). In another study, Wright and colleagues note that medical students identify role models in medical school and that the identification of these role models is powerfully linked with the student's choice of clinical field in residency training (1997). Indeed, a study by Sunita Mutha et al. supports Wright's conclusions and states that "for some of the students, relationship with positive role models had influenced their career specialty choices" (1997, 638), yet they continue to say that "negative role models, in contrast, had strong dissuasive effects on specialty selections. The reported attributes of these individuals included difficult personalities, perceived lack of camaraderie, professional dissatisfaction, and disheartening physician-patient interactions" (1997, 638). Still, in yet another article, Wright et al. (1998) present challenging proof in support of the claim that many physician-teachers do not show the professional characteristics that residents aspire to imitate. Yet nothing guarantees that students will not choose the wrong role model. An emergency department physician who constantly asks her interns to sign her name on every patient who is admitted to the emergency department in order to get an emergency department fee even without her seeing the patient is hardly a good role model. However, to a student whose moral values are still not strong, this might be considered a good role model: she makes good money without really hurting the patients. For others like Brigitte Maheux *et al.*, role models might not be efficient at all (2000). Still, the question that arises here is about the reason behind this lack of professionalism on the part of physician-teachers and the importance of coming up with solutions.[21] Examples of such solutions would be the need to develop a program that develops the moral character of faculty that seem to suffer moral erosion. The reason for this moral erosion will have to be assessed, and the means of addressing it will have to be sorted out through lectures, group discussions, grand rounds, workshops, and the like. Notwithstanding, it remains a fact that human beings can acquire good and bad habits from role models and that one can ultimately learn from both the good and the bad. The good role model remains the *phronimos* to be emulated. *Phronesis* allows for deliberation and judgment in difficult moral situations. In it, intellectual and moral virtues are united. Indeed, one of the criticisms presented against virtue ethics is that it is deficient because it is not *action-guiding*, and that "it lacks the capacity to yield suitably determinate action guides," particularly in new scenarios (Solomon 1988, 432).[22] One can stipulate that it is precisely this crowning virtue that will allow a person (or a physician) to make the choice of action that he must make for the good of the patient. Moreover, considering

---

21. Professionalism here is used in the sense of belonging to a profession and hence making a public promise to do that which is right, to serve the patient, to commit to a life other than self-interest, etc.

22. Further criticism includes leaving its agent to moral luck, being egotistical and concerned only with the agent, and not offering solutions in conflicting cases.

the role of habituation and imitation in the acquisition of habit, is not observing a role model and wanting to emulate her and become somehow another Osler or Peabody in itself action guiding?[23] Also, one can argue that it is precisely when the physician acts, having the ends of medicine in mind, that her virtuous character becomes itself action guiding.

According to Pellegrino and Thomasma, "[t]he power of a faculty model to shape behavior for good or evil is enormous. It far exceeds the power of a lecture or course in ethics. This power generates a serious *de facto* obligation for faculty members and medical schools to be critical of the value systems they express and transmit" (1993, 177). Still, it is my contention that role modeling alone does not suffice. Moral exemplars—be they silent (those who do not speak but simply act) or expressive (those who explain while they act)—are necessary (and indeed indispensable), yet not sufficient for the making of future virtuous physicians. As and Thomasma themselves state, "though the best way to teach virtuous behavior is by example, some significant headway can be made by teaching ethics as a discipline" (1993, 179). Yet "there is no guarantee that a knowledge of ethics itself will make people virtuous" (1993, 179). This issue will be revisited in chapter three.

2.4.2. Organizational Structures and Culture

Medical students do not become virtuous in a vacuum. Learning and habituation take place through participation in an environment where a certain way of professional behavior is modeled, where a certain consistency between word and deed is exhibited. Inconsistencies between word and deed, as in the case of the obstetrician portrayed in chapter one, can have a profound effect on the student, and often function as strong teaching tools that are hard to undo. In addition, virtues and ethics need to be integrated throughout the teaching hospital. Virtues and ethics have to integrally pervade an institution's culture as a system of shared values and beliefs that uphold and promote professionalism or else students will experience a kind of moral and intellectual schizophrenia. *"Do as I say, not as I do"* is not the best way to help neophyte physicians internalize the virtues of a good physician. Physicians, staff, administrators, control systems, the entire bureaucratic structure interact in such a way as to make up the behavioral norms of the institution. As

---

23. Nafsika Athanassoulis argues that the virtuous person is an exemplar and that "[i]f virtue consists of the right reason and the right desire," it will be action-guiding (2006).

Gregory Pence puts it, "[m]orality is not learned the way one learns to play a flute or do a tracheotomy by observing a "master" proficient in a certain craft or technique. Compassion similarly is not learned from a Master of Compassion (or the chief role-model thereof). Instead, it is developed, or not, by the "shape" of the medical environment in which students learn medicine. The overall medical context in which students thrive or stagnate is more important than the efforts (however noble) of any one individual" (Pence 1983, 190). Virtues will have to be nourished by the organization, the mini-society in which students learn and thrive. Ultimately, it is the general culture of the institution that affects everyone and helps mold character, creating a certain ethos particular to an institution. This general ethos engulfs members entirely. Members blend in to the extent that one can recognize to which institution they belong in terms of their ethos. The parts make up the whole, and the whole affects the parts. The institutional structure is responsible for a certain ethical profile precisely because the parts make the whole and the whole assumes an identity of its own which affects the parts. Consequently, minute details count. This is one form of the hidden curriculum of which more will be said in chapter three.

One might contend that the virtues (or vices) of students are already fixed prior to their entering medical school, and hence it is useless to speak of teaching virtues. One might even argue that this talk of teaching the virtues is too idealistic and will not withstand the test of modern times—that is, the question of whether one can be moral in an immoral world. I contend that we cannot and indeed should not afford to be otherwise. Although moral perfection, or complete virtuousness, cannot be achieved, nevertheless it can be set as a framework, a goal to be pursued. Simply because one did not get the Nobel Prize in literature does not mean that one should stop writing. How many students of music give up the piano because they could not master Tchaikovsky's first piano concerto? The closer one gets to the goal, the better one becomes. Whether virtues can or should be taught are two questions answered in the affirmative. The need to teach virtues and to help students internalize them becomes more evident and pressing as studies reveal that often medical students enter medical school with a form of idealism that usually dissipates as they move on from year to year in their medical training. William Branch et al. found that medical students start out with strong empathic identifications with patients, an empathy which leads to respect and compassion (1998). With time, students start experiencing what came to be referred to as "moral erosion." Evidence shows that moral change takes place during medical school although in the wrong direction (Branch 2000; Feudtner et al. 1994; Lind 2000; Sheehan et al., 1990). Moral change, in one direction or the other, illustrates the plasticity of the brain: selected areas in the brain exhibit a mechanism of neurogenesis that continues throughout life, including into old age. Stimulation in the form of an "enriched environment" in aging experimental animals (an environment with a lot of areas including objects to explore and adapt to) enhanced both neurogenesis and performance. Functional Magnetic Resonance Imaging studies on humans have also revealed evidence of plasticity with acquisition of new functions in new areas in a number of situations in adults. Consequently, the view upholding continued plasticity and learning and acquisition is substantiated by scientific data (Tonchev et al., 2003; Abrous et al., 2005; Zhang et al., 2005). Several research studies have been released about this topic. If alterations happen in one direction, they can happen in another.

In this chapter, a brief account of Aristotle's virtue ethics was presented to support the contention that some of the ideas present in Aristotle's *NE* can be used as a guide by medical educators to develop the character of the neophyte physician. The making of the good physician and the shaping of the moral character of the student of medicine was also discussed along with the argument that this can be done by instilling core virtues by means of habituation which will eventually be internalized, thus leading the physician to realizing the ends of medicine and living a happy life. If virtue is to be taught, there need to be role models in medical schools and attention paid to a sustained organizational structure and culture that allow for the development of the virtues. The central question then becomes *how to ensure that change takes place in the right direction and to avoid the moral erosion of future physicians?*

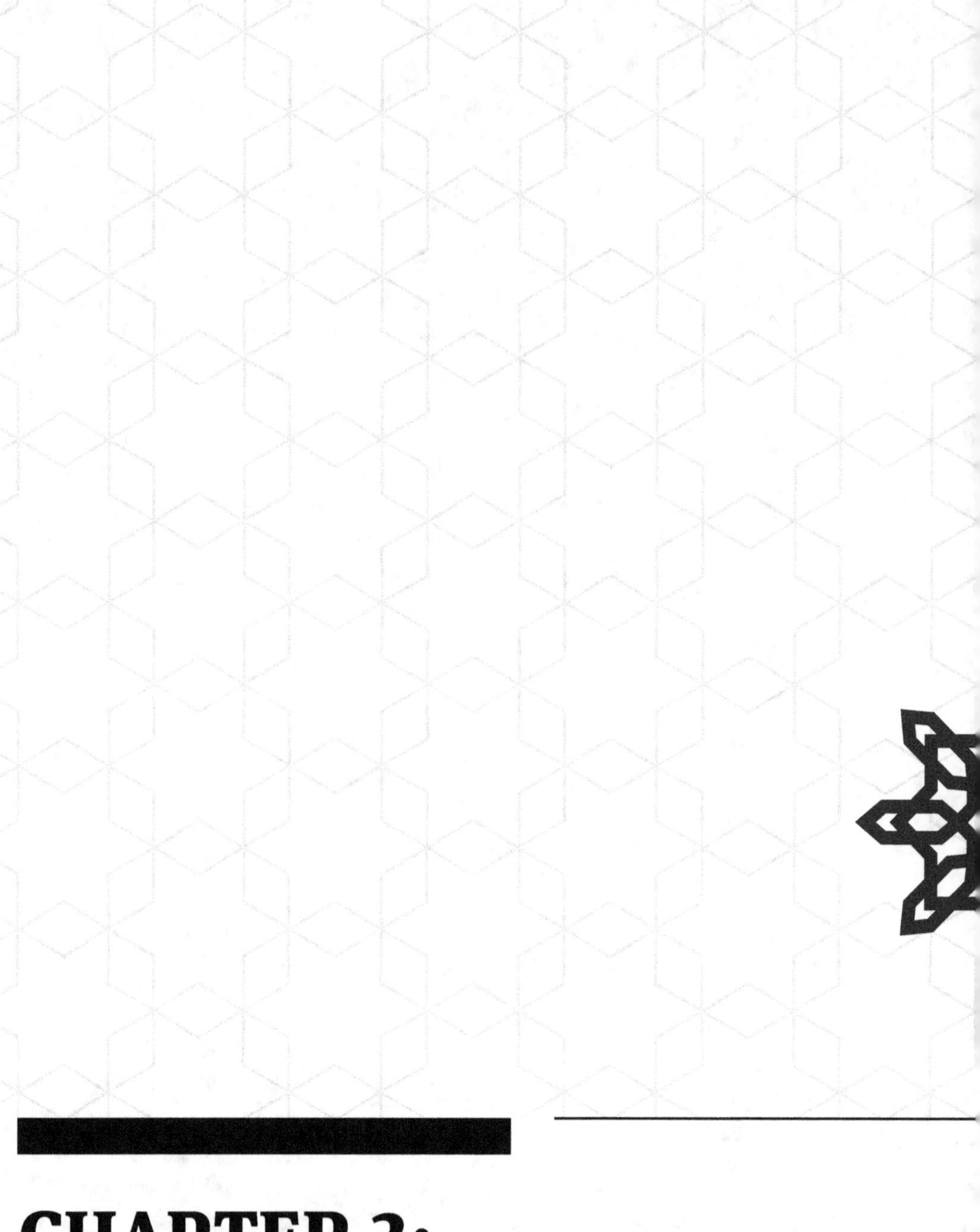

CHAPTER 3:
THE MORAL DEVELOPMENT OF THE MEDICAL STUDENT AND THE CURRICULUM

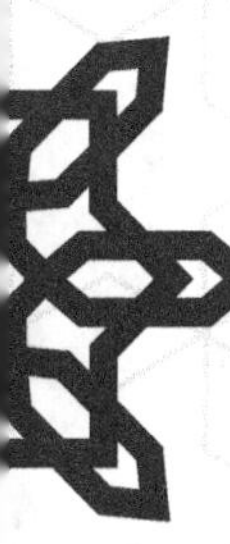

A hidden curriculum is not something one just finds; one must go hunting for it

—J. R. Martin, "What Should We Do with a Hidden Curriculum When We Find One?" (1994, 158)

During their clinical rotations, medical students face a variety of cases that pose ethical dilemmas. Some of these include but are not limited to mistreating patients in the Outpatient Clinic without explaining to them their diagnoses, ordering unnecessary tests, taking photos of anesthetized patients in the operating room without their prior consent, and giving preferential treatment to first-class patients over second- and third-class patients. Ideally, the same service should be provided to all patients, but whether or not they receive it tends to depend on the patients' income and insurance premiums. In the hospital setting, the second- or third-class patient shares a room and therefore pays lower rates for hospital services, while the first-class patient has a private room and pays a higher fee.[1] Medical students often feel as if they are suffering from what I might call "moral schizophrenia"; they are told to behave in one way, but observe attending physicians, whom they are supposed to emulate, behaving in another. These students march enthusiastically into the wards, proud of their white gowns, of what they stand for, only to see that what actually takes place does not always accord with what they have learned in their ethics courses. What will happen to these neophyte physicians if they continue to be inundated with such contradictory experiences? The previous chapter concluded with the question: *how to ensure that change takes place in the right direction and to avoid the moral erosion of future physicians.* This chapter considers the different types of curricula that play a role in the making of the future physician. While it is my contention that the formal curriculum is pivotal in the training of the future physician, I argue that it is not sufficient for forming the virtuous physician. What is called the hidden curriculum is far too important to be neglected since it may play a crucial role in ensuring that changes take place in the right direction and that the moral erosion of future physicians is avoided. Currently, the hidden curriculum has a negative influence on students of medicine who find themselves being taught one thing from the formal curriculum and yet receive different implicit messages from the hidden and informal curricula. Thus, I will start with general definitions of the

---

1. The major difference would be in terms of the fees the patients have to pay at the hospital. The first-class/second-class/third-class categories are mainly for in-house patients. Ideally, the service should not differ, but in reality, it does. Thus, a second-class or third-class patient would pay less for their bed per night at the hospital, and charges for tests and services such as blood tests, X-rays, pathology, and medications also would be less. These patients share a double-occupancy room and bathroom with another patient. It is no different in outpatient clinics. If patients want to be treated by a particular attending physician, they go to private clinics and see whomever they want as long as they can afford the hospital's fixed fees. If they are from a lower socio-economic class, then they go to what is known as the Outpatient Department of a hospital where they are seen first by a resident and then by a faculty member (if they are lucky enough). Here also, the rates for labs and so on are reduced.

different relevant forms of curricula and move on to an analysis of each in an attempt at showing their roles in the making of a future physician. I shall argue that the formal curriculum is wanting, and that medical schools should pay more attention to the informal curriculum if they want to ensure that future physicians will have the necessary character traits that will allow them to *do the right thing even when no one is looking*. In doing so, I will take the example of one particular unit of medical education, namely the physician-patient relationship, frequently emphasized in medical education and ethics courses. I will also argue that a curriculum change alone, both formal and informal, will not work unless organizational changes go hand in hand with this endeavor (an idea already alluded to in chapter two).

3.1. The Curriculum

Medical students matriculate into medical schools in the hope of learning how to become doctors. Most matriculation criteria in Lebanon and the USA are based on the applicants' MCAT scores and their undergraduate grade point averages (GPAs). However, evaluation of suitability for medical school should not be limited to academic capabilities because one can be academically successful yet suffer from a lack of moral qualities or, worse, show evidence of bad moral judgement. Jordan Cohen, president of the Association of American Medical Colleges in 2002, expresses these concerns:

> *. . . the imbalance that currently exists in how we convey to applicants the selection criteria we use. I'm referring, of course, to our tendency to underemphasize, because they are harder to measure, the personal characteristics we are seeking in our applicants and to overemphasize the more easily measured indices of academic achievement (Cohen 2002, 476–477).*

He goes on to challenge the medical community to "help devise better tools for evaluating students' personal characteristics" (2002, 477). Indeed, according to Penny Salvatori (2001), there is enough evidence in the literature that the performance of students in the first two pre-clinical years of medical school is sufficiently predicted by these purely academic scores. Medical schools offer a variety of curricula that aim at graduating skilled physicians, all having in common a core curriculum in basic and clinical sciences. Still, Robert Murden et al. (1978) and W. T. Basco et al. (2000) find a strong enough correlation between non-cognitive measures and clinical performance to make one ponder the importance (and possibility) of assessing character traits in medical school admissions, assuming it can be done. As mentioned in chapter one, there are myriad character traits that medical schools deem desirable in physicians, and these are often qualities that reflect a school's mission and objectives as well as its culture (Albanese et al. 2003; Reiter and Eva 2005). Yet, in the absence of criteria to assess such qualities, what is to be done? Should all students of medicine who matriculate be allowed to graduate if they meet the curricular requirements? Or should their ethical behavior and character also be factors in their qualification to graduate? A study revealed that cheating in medical school is linked to cheating later on (Tolkin and Glick 2007). Jeremy Laurance reported on a medical student who cheated during her final examination but was allowed to graduate "despite being caught red-handed" (Laurance 2000). In an editorial in *The Western Journal of Medicine,* "MSMW" states that frequent cheaters are likely to be incorrigible, and that "[i]n the professional and public interest, these should be exposed and expelled from the school or from the profession, even at the expense of the time-consuming and costly legal actions that are almost certain to ensue" (MSMW 1982, 145). That author went on to argue that less frequent cheaters should be educated and counseled. In an editorial in the same journal (1982, 77), A. Lasnover recounts a story that made him pessimistic about cheating and its effect beyond medical school after witnessing a fellow doctor forging signatures that entitled visitors at a scientific and commercial exhibit to enter a drawing to win a portable television set. Lasnover concludes by saying, "[M]y experience leads me to doubt the conclusions stated in your editorial. I shudder to think that whereas only a small number of our colleagues behave in such fashion, the numbers may increase in the future" (1982 77).

How should a medical school handle cheaters? Should students caught cheating be allowed to continue in medical school? Should one accept applicants who have that character flaw to begin with? Can this flaw (in its varying degrees) be assessed from the beginning, prior to admission? Can one build up moral fiber in a matriculant who lacks it? These are important questions. The curriculum, in its several components and kinds, plays an important part in managing them.

What is a curriculum, to begin with? It is not easy to find a clear and comprehensive definition of this widely used term. While Hugh Sockett warned his readers: "Seek not for any definition of curriculum. There is no such elixir" (Sockett 1976, 88), Beauchamp attempted to define it, saying that a curriculum is "a written plan depicting the scope and arrangement of the projected educational program for a school" (Beauchamp 1982, 25). Lawrence Stenhouse, on the other hand, gave a holistic explanation and argued that a curriculum is "everything that is happening in the classroom, department, Faculty or School, or the University as a whole" (Stenhouse 1975, 2). David Kern et al. (1998) define a curriculum as "a planned educational experience" (1998, 1) and Alan Rogers argued that:

> *[T]he curriculum is often seen as a body of knowledge, the content of education to which the students need to be exposed. But curriculum is much wider than a list of subjects to be studied; it is not only what you say but how you say it! Curriculum is all the planned experiences to which the learner may be exposed in order to achieve the learning goals (Rogers 1996, 176).*

Notwithstanding these definitions (or lack thereof), the curriculum is much more than what is presented in the classroom by the faculty. It extends far beyond the classroom to encompass what is not said or taught. The curriculum can be said to include everything that occurs in the medical school and more. Thus, the curriculum in medical school is like a fine Persian carpet: one incorrect loop can impair its quality and beauty. Consequently, no one will buy it. In addition, it will damage the reputation of the entire Persian carpet industry.

Leslie Owen Wilson, a professor of education at the University of Wisconsin – Stevens Point, listed and defined eleven curriculum types among which are the curriculum-in-use (formal), the informal, the societal, and the phantom (Wilson 2005).[2] There have been efforts in the last decades to reassess the medical curricula, with their traditional emphasis on basic sciences and clinical medicine, and to add a number of bioethics courses in the hope that they will help shape the moral compass of students and sculpt their moral fiber.[3]

A few years back, a physician at Johns Hopkins said: "Today, doctors are both more powerful and more deaf. They are far less helpless in the face of suffering, yet they often cannot hear the cries that evoke no possibility of remedy. A more humanistic education might heal the physician's deafness" (Overby 2005, 25–26). Mastery of

---

2. The url for this information is no longer active. The information was moved to the author's personal blog, and can be found at https://thesecondprinciple.com/instructional-design/.

3. It is important to note that I am not advocating indoctrination, which is detrimental to healthy thought. Indoctrination involves the blind absorption of virtues while inculcation entails accepting them with reflection and critical thinking, and eventually adopting them because one is convinced that they are right and good. The phronimos reflects and thinks before making a decision.

technical skills and scientific knowledge are necessary to becoming a good physician, but they are not sufficient. Doctors and the public are becoming more aware of the moral expectations of physicians, and the public is becoming more and more disenchanted with physicians' morals, as noted in chapter one. The American Medical Association has emphasized the importance of teaching ethics and has developed a unit for its teaching, and the General Medical Council of England has identified ethical behavior as a crucial component of education. The British "Pond Report" (Institute of Medical Ethics 1987) has endorsed the integration of a broad course in medical ethics within the curricula of British medical schools and has recommended that "time should be set aside within existing teaching for ethical reflection" (Gillon 1987, 115). Ethics teaching has become part of integrated medical curricula in recent years because of the belief that such training plays a role in the shaping of character. These programs have more or less similar goals, described by Steven Miles et al. as aiming to "develop physicians' values, social perspectives, and interpersonal skills for the practice of medicine" (1989, 705). Modern schools of medicine are resorting to modern styles of teaching. Some have recourse to computer-based teaching and audiovisual aids to exemplify the importance of virtues. The movie *The Doctor*, based on the memoir of real life surgeon Ed Rosenbaum and entitled *A Taste of My Own Medicine*, is one example.[4] This is all part of the formal curriculum.

3.1.1. The Formal Curriculum and the Making of a Good Physician

The formal curriculum is the declared and usually written curriculum, defined by UNESCO's education department as "the planned programme of objectives, content, learning experiences, resources and assessment offered by a school. It is sometimes called the 'official curriculum'" (UNESCO 2010). The guiding principle of offering ethics in the formal curriculum is that, as a discipline, ethics plays a role in high-quality patient care and professional behavior. In 1910, Abraham Flexner, to whom the change in twentieth-century medical education is owed, maintained that in contemporary life the medical profession is an organ distinguished by society for its highest goals, rather than a business that one should exploit (Flexner 1910). The same can be said of the medical profession today. In the US, in general and at the time of the Flexner Report, several medical schools were proprietary schools that prioritized profit over education. Following Flexner's report, the change was made

---

4. The movie portrays a doctor who cares little for the emotional and psychological well-being of patients. As the movie unfolds, we see him diagnosed with a tumor. At this point, the change begins, and he metamorphoses from an arrogant physician to one who cares for his patients and teaches his students to do the same.

towards a medical education that emphasized strong biomedical sciences along with hands-on clinical training in an attempt at graduating skilled medical practitioners. Notwithstanding, Flexner did not overlook the humane face of medicine. In addition to the fundamental sciences, he referred to the indispensable insight and sympathy of physicians and acknowledged that scientific progress has tremendously modified their ethical responsibility (Flexner 1910). We find the same idea echoed years later with Pellegrino (1974), who argued that while skill and craft are essential to the physician, they are not enough. For Pellegrino, without humanism, physicians are deficient practitioners. Today, the revolution ahead of us is one that aims at graduating skilled physicians with a sense of morals because this is precisely where the inefficiencies lie. Yet formal education (in communication skills and bioethics, among other subjects), alone, will not make students morally better physicians. Nowadays, students of medicine as well as physicians are faced with myriad ethical concerns during their medical training and practice. These include disagreements among patients, relatives, and healthcare professionals over treatment options; difficulties in obtaining informed consent; medical error; confidentiality; and more. As such, it is often argued that students of medicine should be well trained in clinical ethics, and that practicing physicians should have at least a minimum level of ethical sensitivity and critical analysis that allows them to deal with complex cases. In an attempt at ensuring that, most medical schools around the world have introduced courses and programs in bioethics which include lectures on the nature of moral discourse and on moral theories. However, students of medicine often remark that there is a gap between the theories offered in ethics and the concrete moral dilemmas they face in the wards. Thus, questions and statements like "how will deontology help me decide on whether the life of the baby is more important than that of the mother?" or "ethics is great, but really, it is a theoretical exercise that has no practical bearing for me" are becoming catchphrases that often reverberate in bioethics courses. This problem has become less pervasive as case studies have started being used in an attempt to add to the abstract theories taught to medical students, hoping thereby to enhance their ethical reasoning and moral sensitivity. Nevertheless, these vignettes are mostly presented as an addendum to a unit or a theory, often engaging the students only temporarily and not leaving room for a convincing rational conclusiveness, as many details are left out of the picture. Such absent details can be vital in assisting the decision-maker to weigh the relevant considerations of a case. Students leave the debate confused, often forgetful if not skeptical of ethics and its relevance. In an attempt at remedying this, several modes of ethics teaching have been introduced to the formal curriculum: lectures, seminars, case-based analysis, debates, and problem-based learning (Parker 1995; Tysinger et al. 1997); role play (Nelson and Eliastam 1991); and narrative ethics (Jones 1999). Teaching in the formal curriculum entails professors consciously acting as good role models, using deliberate reflection, and conveying accounts that involve patients, doctors, staff, and other members of the healthcare team. These attempts may make some students more ethically sensitive to a number of issues but will not necessarily induce them to act in the right way. Thus, a student can learn that he ought to respect autonomy yet may actually choose to override it. One can know how to respectfully greet a patient, yet still act with arrogance. In other words, the emphasis in ethics courses is rather on teaching students the skill of identifying and analyzing moral problems in order to solve them. However, something else is needed to bridge the gap between theory and practice that will impel the student to behave in a certain way and to be a certain kind of person. Pellegrino discusses seven questions he encountered from critics relating to the teaching of medical ethics. As to whether teaching medical ethics makes a difference (1989, 701), Pellegrino answers that no proven link exists between ethics and the teaching of basic sciences and clinical behavior, and thus ethics should not be singled out in that respect. Yet, he does refer to a study (Pellegrino et al. 1985) which revealed that physicians who took courses in ethics "perceived themselves better prepared to make the ethical decisions they confronted in daily practice" (1989, 701). As to whether ethics can be taught, he acquiesced, although he noted that the teaching of ethics is not "expected to guarantee virtue" (1989, 702). Moreover, and perhaps what is even more serious, is that students often witness the physicians who teach them the precepts necessary for good behavior subsequently violate those precepts themselves. A typical example is a case reported by a student in his second year of medical school in a renowned teaching hospital who was shadowing one of the physicians for over an hour. He came back flabbergasted at the physician's poor communication skills and insensitivity towards the patients he had been seeing, and particularly for the physician's not giving the patients enough time and for making sure to ask every patient to pay the bill when abruptly announcing the end of the visit. What shocked the student even more was that this physician was the one who taught the communication skills course and who served for some time on several ethics-related committees.

It can be argued that past incidents of ethical infractions and misconduct as well as negative consequences of misusing and abusing the rapid development in biotechnology could be avoided if neophyte students of medicine were given courses or had proper instruction in bioethics. This is a legitimate claim, to some extent, if one is willing to argue that the past mishaps would not have happened had the culprit been aware of proper ethical conduct and of major ethical theories. Yet, I contend that this argument does not hold. Typical examples can be taken from the realm of research ethics: the Nuremberg Code, which marked the beginning of human subject protection and was the basis for human subject research ethics, actually came about as a consequence of war crimes and the resulting Nuremberg trials in 1945–1946. It did not prevent scientists from breaking research ethics standards, as evident in the well-known Willowbrook hepatitis experiments carried out on mentally challenged children in New York State in 1956. More recently, after the prominent Belmont Report of 1979, we have witnessed several infractions such as the Jesse Gelsinger gene experiment at the University of Pennsylvania in 2000 and the Johns Hopkins "Mechanisms of Deep Inspiration-Induced Airway Relaxation Study" (Steinbock, 2002), which led to the death of a volunteer, Ellen Roche, in 2001. Unless one is willing to contend (and prove) that the persons involved in the above-mentioned infractions were oblivious to any ethical constructs, then one should be willing to acknowledge that much more than simple knowledge of ethics is needed to ensure that one does the right thing. Consequently, perhaps a new report (in the tradition of Flexner) should be developed advocating change in medical education. The need for a major redesign of the content of medical training is becoming more pressing with time, particularly with rapid developments in medical technology. However, curricular reform is never uncomplicated or trouble-free, as there are always problems to be envisaged and territorial battles to be anticipated. Thus, the challenge lies in incorporating content into the curriculum in a way that emphasizes its weight relative to other core curricular content. This ties in with the issue of organizational culture, referred to in chapter two, which I will shortly address. Nevertheless, there are many efforts in that direction (Anon 1984; Education Committee of the General Medical Council 1993; General Medical Council 1998; Mennin and Kalishman 1998; Davis et al. 2001; Pascoe et al. 2004). Indeed, according to Herbert Swick et al., among the 116 responding US medical schools he studied, 89.7% reported giving some formal training related to professionalism (Swick et al. 1999).[5] Yet, they argue that "the strategies used to achieve that goal appear inadequate" (1999, 832). Thus, a challenge lies in finding the appropriate faculty and means to teach the revised curriculum.

Consider the following case: M is a medical student in her third year and is currently rotating through the floors. As part of her medical curriculum, she is required to take

---

5. Often defined as the behavior of physicians and how they act during their interactions with patients and society.

a bioethics course that runs through the entire academic year. Thrilled at having the chance to work in the emergency department, she witnesses an incident in which theory clashes with practice. A thirteen-year-old boy limps into the emergency department, aided by his father. The father explains that his son sustained an injury to his ankle while playing soccer. They want to be reassured that his ankle was not fractured. He had been charged a substantial fee upon entering the emergency department and is a self-payer with no insurance. The student examines the patient with the resident-in-charge. The ankle is swollen and very tender, indicating a possible fracture, so they request an X-ray. She prints the request paper and is about to ask the father to get it stamped by the cashier when she is intercepted by the attending physician, who asks her about the case. After she explains the case to him, he gives her a pinkish piece of paper representing an additional and exorbitant fee "that he never fails to give to every single patient." The patient's father objects, and the medical student has to reply that it is the attending physician's fee although the latter had not seen the patient. There are too many situations like this one that make one wonder about the effectiveness of the formal curriculum (in terms of time and content) in helping shape the character of students. Yet, there is almost no proof that the different pedagogical interventions used, however varied and creative they are, change behavior, inducing a physician to act more ethically (Boon and Turner 2004; Tamblyn et al. 2007). This is not to say that the formal courses offered are useless; after all, almost all students who have taken an ethics course are aware of the principles of medical ethics, take into consideration the autonomy of patients, and make an effort to factor in the principles whenever faced with conflicts in the wards. The question is: how deeply ingrained in their character has ethics become? Osler saw the importance of linking character to medicine and spoke to his students about the profession of medicine being unique among others:

> *You are in this profession as a calling, not as a business; as a calling which exacts from you at every turn self-sacrifice, devotion, love and tenderness to your fellow-men. Once you get down to a purely business level, your influence is gone and the true light of your life is dimmed. You must work in the missionary spirit, with a breadth of charity that raises you far above the petty jealousies of life (Osler 1907).*

Some might argue that medicine suffers from the absence of a codified Oslerian presence. Yet, this is not the case since we know that Percival wrote a formal treatise, dedicated to this son (1803), laying down what he called the "code of institutes and precepts" for the professional conduct of physicians. Lessons and lectures in ethics do have a role to play, but to many they are far from able to capture the complexities of ethical life in the wards or to leave a long-lasting imprint on the character of the physician-to-be. Authentic education cannot happen if students are taught one thing during lectures but witness the opposite during rounds. The result may be a kind of cynicism or a process of moral erosion, a decline in moral reasoning during medical school years, as shown by William Branch (1998) and others discussed below.

3.1.1.1. Medical School and Moral Erosion

Students matriculate into medical school with one form or another of ethical self. Some contend that students start medical school imbued with idealism, a strong sense of empathy, and a tendency to identify with patients (Branch 1998). This empathy may serve as "a bulwark against the emotional erosion of difficult times to come" (1998, 362). Branch maintains that students of medicine "feel trapped between the need to live according to their moral principles and the many perceived pressures to suppress their principles in order to fit in as team members" (Branch 2000, 504). Many would agree with this. Still, one question remains: if principles change, were they even principles to begin with? Or were they accidental characteristics attached to the self of the person holding them? The assumption is that principles, once acquired, are there to stay; they are not accidental, a function of context and suitability. A study by Chris Feudtner et al. on the perception of medical students a propos the ethical dilemmas they face during their medical training revealed that certain dilemmas influence students and are detrimental to their moral progress (Feudtner et al. 1994, 670–679). These include observing unethical behavior by other team members, trying to be good team players and not daring to rock the boat, being evaluated by means of grades, developing closer relationships with patients than with the rest of the team, and being slyly coerced to put oneself at risk of personal injury, such as skipping universal precautions whilst carrying out a procedure (1994, 670). The study reports one student saying: "Slowly I'm seeing my classmates become 'destroyed' and it scares me! I've become so cynical that it's just not right!!" (1994, 675). The authors conclude that ethical education as presently taught is "ineffectual" and that what is needed is the fostering of ethical standards (1994, 678). Another study by Thomas Wolf et al. revealed that "developmental stressors" of medical education affect students (Wolf et al. 1989, 19–23). Jack Coulehan and Pamela Williams contend that, as they matriculate into medical school, students are "good seeds," but "the lack of nourishment and the exposure to defoliants they encounter in medical training . . . alter [their] beliefs and value systems so that a 'commitment to the well-being of others' either withers or turns into something barely recognizable" (Coulehan and Williams 2001, 599). In their longitudinal study on erosion, Mohammadreza Hojat et al. came to the conclusion that "the escalation of cynicism and atrophy of idealism has long been recognized as part of students' socialization in medical school and their adaptation to a professional role. This downward trend has also been observed in the ethical erosion of medical students during their clinical training" (Hojat et al. 2009, 1189). They conclude by saying that "profound changes to enhance empathy during medical education should be considered by leaders in medical education [as] a mandate, not an option, if the public is to be served in the best possible manner" (2009, 1190). Obviously, medical education plays a role in shaping medical students' characters. Some have argued that it is dehumanizing, inflexible, discouraging, and, at times, offensive and abusive (Pfifferling 1980; Sliver 1982; Weinstein 1983; Rosenberg and Silver 1984). Indeed, studies have revealed that abuse of medical students—verbal or otherwise, such as embarrassment, intimidation, and undermining of self-esteem— can be among the more seriously traumatic and upsetting, let alone demoralizing, characteristics of medical education (Silver 1982; Rosenberg and Silver 1984). The study by Wolf et al. revealed that most students saw themselves as becoming more cynical during their education years (1989, 20). They also reported that they developed concerns with making money. John Testerman et al. speak of a process of "traumatic deidealization": the professional socialization experienced in medical school that leads students of medicine to develop a sense of cynicism (Testerman et al. 1996, S43). The authors speak of two models that explain the rise of this cynicism: the first is the "intergenerational transmission" model, where cynicism is seen as a learned response to abusive behavior and maltreatment from superiors, and the second is the "professional identity" model. The latter is explained as a temporary product of the harsher aspects of the professional socialization process. Here the student fights to build his identity in an environment filled with challenges and ethically dubious constructs (1996, S43). The authors conclude that "[m]edical students begin their training with altruistic motives and idealized concepts of health. As inexperienced and powerless members of the healthcare team, however, students may develop cynicism as a means to manage their environment" (1993, S45). Thus, we now speak of the pre-cynical years rather than the pre-clinical years. Authentic education does not happen if professors argue for the importance of ethics while the organization does not worry about putting it into practice. Bruce Newton et al. argue that the results of their study imply that student empathy is influenced by medical education and that medical students become immunized against humanistic values after they matriculate into medical school (Newton et al. 2008, 244–249). Here comes the importance of what I call the "clandestine curricula" and what medical sociologist Frederic Hafferty (1998) has designated more specifically as the "hidden curriculum" and the "informal curriculum."

3.1.2. The Clandestine Curricula

The issue of curricular reform is becoming more important every day. This is especially so with rapid developments in medical technology and ensuing ethical issues, which, in turn, make biomedical ethics an important topic that can no longer be brushed aside. Bioethics is no longer a luxury; increasingly it is becoming a core subject in many medical schools. Yet, much of what is learned is taught indirectly, outside the formal curricula that medical schools profess to teach.

The teaching milieu, in general and, for our purposes, in medical schools, consists of a number of different yet interrelated elements. At the center, there is the observed and clearly stated curriculum, generally known as the formal curriculum. Yet, there are also two other areas with equal, if not greater, impact: the hidden curriculum and the informal curriculum. These are clandestine curricula, yet they exert enormous power on the teaching and learning environments of a medical school. According to Hafferty, the hidden curriculum is the "set of influences that function at the level of organizational structure and culture" (1998, 404), whereas the informal curriculum is an "unscripted, predominantly ad hoc, and highly interpersonal form of teaching and learning that takes place among and between faculty and students" (1998, 404). It is my contention that the hidden and the informal curricula play a much more crucial role in the making of the physician than the formal one. Indeed, I will even venture to argue that the informal curriculum can either undo or enforce much of what the formal curriculum teaches.

3.1.3. The Hidden Curriculum

The hidden curriculum consists of the unnoticed set of influences working alongside the structure and culture of the teaching and learning milieu. According to Alan Cribb and Sarah Bignold, the hidden curriculum summarizes the "processes, pressures and constraints which fall outside of, or are imbedded within, the formal curriculum, and which are often unarticulated or unexplored" (1999, 197). Hence, medical education turns out to be a cultural concept affected by societal factors and internal belief systems. The term "hidden curriculum" is said to have been coined by Philip Jackson (1968), who argued that in order to succeed in schools, students must learn to conform to the formal and informal rules of the school, which include beliefs and attitudes propagated through a process of socialization. The same applies to medical schools. Students learn by being exposed to hidden messages often propagated by the institution, and this is precisely why the medical school is viewed as a moral community where everything matters and has consequences. Thus, it matters how rules are framed, policies are drafted, walls are decorated, and residents and physicians walk, talk, and dress. It all has an effect on the making of the future physician. Walking can be a lesson in humility or in arrogance; talking, a lesson in modesty or high-handedness; dressing, a lesson in reticence and cleanliness, or in showing-off and messiness. It is all about what kind of physician one ought to become, and this is strongly related to the hidden lessons and the hidden curricula, as nothing happens in a vacuum. This is precisely why a very thin line separates the hidden curriculum from the informal one. Notwithstanding, one important matter of concern to the hidden curriculum is what the medical institution claims it cares about when it introduces formal courses in ethics and what actually happens at the level of the organization.

3.1.4. Curriculum Development, the Hidden Curriculum, and Organizational Culture

Instilling a culture of ethics in medical school cannot happen if the organizational culture of that school does not encourage ethics. To work on curriculum development with ethics as a major component means that the organizational environment of the school must support this newly emergent culture, otherwise it will not survive. This calls for a paradigm shift that needs to happen slowly and smoothly, or else will backfire. To Thomas Kuhn (1996), a paradigm is an exemplar that demonstrates a rule, a sort of an archetype worthy of imitation. In Kuhn's historical perspective, the development of scientific thought does not occur in a simple linear progression where one idea is built on others until a specific agreed-upon conclusion is reached. Instead, there is often a kind of rivalry of hypotheses and theories held by different groups or schools of thought. One paradigm may be dominant until it runs into difficulty. This is what is happening in medical schools. The prevalence of an organizational structure that undercuts ethics is no longer viable, as there exist significant anomalies that cannot be satisfactorily explained within the constructs of the paradigm. Some medical schools survive on competing paradigms that cannot survive for long, as each paradigm answers some, but not all of the questions that contemporary issues force onto the scene. Hence, no one of the competing paradigms is capable of asserting absolute authority in the field. Eventually, a paradigm shift will have to occur.

It is my contention that a paradigm shift needs to occur in the direction of an organizational change towards a culture of ethics. This is so for a very simple reason: medical schools and medical doctors have reached a point where they cannot afford to set aside issues pertaining to bioethics. Such issues have become ingrained in the everyday dealings of physicians: patient care, social care, insurance companies, physician-physician relationships, professionalism, and research, to mention but a few. If medicine is to thrive and remain a "profession," a clear culture of ethics will have to be shaped, gradually but firmly.

According to Edgar Schein, an organizational culture is "a system of shared meaning held by members that distinguishes the organization from other organizations" (1983, 32). He argues that the vision of the organization's founders has a deep impact on the organization's culture, and organizational efficacy is possible only when there is harmony between the mission of an organization and its culture. Yet, when the culture itself is becoming one where ethics cannot be brushed aside any longer, where physicians are being questioned for their lack of good character and virtuousness, so to speak, something ought to happen at the level of the organization, or otherwise endeavors for change are bound to fail. Organizational culture is a powerful determinant of the behavior of the people in an organization. It involves what the school professes it does—its formal declarations, its practices, its policies and procedures, and the way it manages its affairs on a daily basis. Organizational culture plays a vital role in an organization's success in achieving its mission and objectives, which in schools of medicine includes the making of good and ethical physicians.[6] Thus, an organizational virtue ethics is a key aspect of a fully developed ethics of virtue for medicine. Henceforth, the organizational structure of the institution, which to date has remained as it was ever since the Flexnerian revolution, needs to change if the mission statement of the school in graduating excellent physicians with humane and high ethical standards is to be met. What does such a

---

6. Cf. chapter two.

change involve? To begin with, it involves a change at the level of the mentality of an institution's employees. Bioethics should no longer be perceived as something supplemental to the practice of medicine, but as something inherent and inseparable from the practice itself. There needs to be a written code of ethics of conduct for all students, faculty members, staff, and other related professionals, and this code needs to be enforced, or else it will be useless.[7] Compliance standards need to be enforced with responses to offences and assurance that they will not recur. At this point, the nature of rewards becomes relevant. A medical school that bestows a "Scientist of the Year" award should also start thinking of bestowing something similar to a "Humanism Award." All medical school employees should undergo periodic professional development training in ethics akin to what is required from continuing medical education programs. This will allow professionals to stay abreast of new developments in medical ethics and keep them attuned to the fact that medicine and ethics can no longer be considered as separate, but rather that medicine is a moral endeavor. A mechanism of consultation and advice regarding matters pertaining to professionalism and ethics as well as a mechanism for confidential reporting needs to be established. Thus, it should be well understood that medicine is a moral enterprise and that being virtuous is not a plus, but a minimum requirement of all those who are involved in the care of patients. Most importantly, there should be a commitment on the part of those at the top of the hierarchy, and this must be reflected in the school's mission statement as well as its policies and procedures. Finally, it is important to note that the practices of those in prominent positions need to be in line with the new emergent culture of ethics. The behavior of superiors and peers in addition to formal organizational policies are highly influential. Furthermore, one has to ensure that there are no contradictions, as contradictions in the culture of an organization obstruct change and hinder ethical progress. For example, scrutiny should be exercised on white coat ceremonies; committees;[8] required and elective courses; how resources are allocated; what awards are granted, if at all, and for what achievements; which courses are better equipped; what kinds of pictures or photos decorate the walls of a teaching hospital; dress codes; and other similar issues that are part of the hidden curriculum and affect the making of the physician-to-be. Such minor issues have a great impact on the hidden curriculum and carry hidden messages. A discussion of the white coat ceremony will follow, as it represents a major curricular event of growing importance.

---

7. See my discussion on p. 36 and p. 44 concerning the interplay between action-based and character-based approaches to ethics.

8. For example, oversight of the role, work, and impact of the health ethics committee.

To contend that it is enough to have virtuous physicians and that organizations do not matter is, in a way, psychologically insensitive and morally flawed. Thus, when those in power, at the top of the hierarchy, overlook their moral responsibilities, the expected result will be some form of demise of the profession as defined in terms of its ends.

3.1.4.1. White Coat Ceremonies

In ancient times and until the nineteenth century, physicians used to wear black, the color of formal attire, as medical encounters were thought of as formal occasions. Symbolically, the color black also denoted that medicine was not always capable of helping a patient, and its practice also was considered synonymous with quackery and worthless cures (Shryock, 1947). Practitioners were painted clad in black, as in the famous *The Gross Clinic* by American artist Thomas Eakins; that work depicts an amphitheatre at the Jefferson Medical College, where Dr. Gross and his assistants, all in black, operate on a patient. Interestingly, a decade or so later, in *The Agnew Clinic*, the same painter portrays physicians, assistants, and patients all clothed in white, denoting cleanliness, purity, and hygiene. The shift in medical attire took place within a brief period, and black was discarded for white. The effect of the white coat became so pervasive that many pediatricians and psychiatrists now choose not to wear them in order not to affect their patients. Recent literature warns against the "white coat syndrome," a condition during which patients become anxious in the presence of a medical practitioner in white, manifested by high blood pressure, and gives advice on how to avoid it.

White coat ceremonies are relatively recent in medical schools and are often viewed as a curricular event. In addition to some of its practical purposes, such as protecting physicians from obvious contamination, the white coat stands as a reminder to physicians of their professional duties as set down by Hippocrates, who ordained them to lead their lives and practice their art in honor and decency. In 1993, in conformity with the Hippocratic spirit, the Arnold P. Gold Foundation of Columbia University College of Physicians and Surgeons instigated a white coat ceremony that has since been adopted by several medical schools. According to Dr. Gold, a pediatric neurologist, students of medicine were failing to espouse humanism and professionalism. This led him and his wife to establish the Gold Foundation, which supported the institution of the white coat ceremony. According to David Stern and Maxine Papadakis, this ceremony is an event during which students "learn the meaning of the responsibility that comes with wearing a white coat, the expectations for humanism and professionalism" (2006, 1794). To Arnold Gold, the white coat symbolizes the medical profession of 1954, when:

> *. . . there were none of the competing values and messages that are prevalent today. Residents and students did what their attendings modeled. Altruism was the rule, and meeting the needs of the patients, whatever the personal cost, was the norm. In effect, both the formal and the hidden curriculum were one in the same, and expectations for success were clearly defined (2006, 546).*

The white coat ceremony is regarded as a "rite of passage, welcoming the new medical student into the medical profession, albeit as a medical student" (Gillon 2000, 83). During such ceremonies, medical students are welcomed by the school's administration, lectured about the virtues of the humane physician and the symbolism of the white coat, and asked to recite the Hippocratic Oath and promise to practice medicine in compassion and humility and to follow humane and moral standards, all in the presence of family members and guests. They then don their white coats, now recognized as a prominent symbol of the medical profession. The Gold Foundation explicates the white coat ceremony as an experience which "emphasizes the importance of compassionate care for the patient as well as scientific proficiency" (The Arnold P. Gold Foundation 2013). Raanan Gillon, who began by being skeptical about the ceremony, as he himself admits (2000, 84), avers that he has changed his mind and become an enthusiastic supporter, and recommends that all medical schools start introducing a white coat ceremony (2000, 84). With time, the white coat ceremony has become an important tenet of many medical schools, falling within the realm of the hidden curriculum. It not only teaches the physician about the kind of behavior she owes to her future patients, but also indicates that she is in possession of powers and privileges that are not to be abused, and that she belongs to a distinctive profession. The coat, so to speak, impels her to bond with all members of the profession, wherever they are. Yet, the white coat of the twenty-first century is no longer the same white coat of 1954, as presented by Arnold Gold, nor are white coat ceremonies challenge free: patients often confer status and power to those wearing the white coat, and students easily sense that. Once wearing the white coat, the medical student does not necessarily feel covered by a garment of compassion, but rather by one of power, a status earned by the mere fact of wearing the coat. Then the white coat ceremony becomes a double-edged sword and makes one wonder whether this part of the hidden curriculum might not have backfired.[9] If so, what can one do about it? Some students fail to recognize that it is not the white coat that makes them, but rather, they who make the white coat, and that this relates to character development and to upholding certain values that the white coat is meant to reflect. Indeed, Delese Wear argues that the white coat ceremony may stand in the way of students developing skills of self- reflection that are crucial to the development of virtues and essential to the practice of medicine (1988). She worries about whether the "ceremony, or the white coat itself, is the best vehicle through which to encourage compassionate and humble caregiving" (1998, 735) and suggests alternatives, "new rituals" (1998, 736), that would allow students to see the perspectives of underprivileged and unfortunate people. For example, she suggests instituting "first Fridays" during which students would spend time on the first Friday of each month in community service, on scheduled visits to adult daycare centers, rape crisis centers, community drug boards, and other similar activities. Wear asserts that "first Fridays" could become "the symbol of professional development, a ritualized demonstration of humane medicine, sanctioned by the educators who seek to promote such traits, modeled by caregivers on location, and serving communities whose needs and opinions are often overlooked by the dominant (including the medical) perspectives of our culture" (1998, 737).

In his "Deconstructing the White Coat" (1989), William Branch considers such activities as "first Fridays" and white coat ceremonies. According to him:

> *White coat ceremonies seem to try to inoculate students against the unsavory effects of the informal curriculum: the lack of compassion, the blurring of ethical boundaries, the treating of patients like objects, and other moral quagmires that probably affect the education of medical students at least as powerfully as the hidden curriculum of symbols does (1989, 741).*

Branch concludes that white coat ceremonies and "first Fridays" are "inadequate to support the professional moral and ethical development of students" (1989, 741). He adds that while Wear's proposal is praiseworthy, it might lead to cynicism unless its realization is cautiously designed and backed up by suitable construct and mentoring. In 1995, Branch and his colleagues came up with an alternative approach to support the professional development of third-year medical students (1998, 741):

---

9. This also explains much of the grievance felt by medical students when told that as students they will be wearing short coats, denoting their status as students, instead of the regular ones the actual doctors wear.

a "required curriculum of weekly small-group sessions in which students reflected on their ethical and humanistic values throughout the third-year clerkships" (1989, 742). Although this alternative does offer students an opportunity to keep their moral values active during their clerkship years, it yet remains a fact that the exercise belongs to the realm of the formal curriculum, and one can argue that inherent in both proposals—those of Wear and Branch—is a tacit worry about the creation of a virtuous physician. The hidden curriculum and the informal curriculum are here to stay and have powerful impacts on students and faculty alike. They lurk within the organizational culture of the institution regardless of whether one wants them, is aware of them, or is attuned to them. Thus, *Branch* concludes his deconstruction of the white coat by saying that there ought to be more white coat ceremonies (1998, 741).

It is my contention that a white coat ceremony is just a medium: what is significant is what happens *during* this ceremony. What message is being conveyed? Who is giving a speech, and what does it say? Who is donning the white coat? Does this person have the characteristics of a role model worthy of emulation? Is the white coat ceremony still-born, or will its significance hold strong regardless? What is the hidden message conveyed to the physician-to-be? Is it that ethics matters and is an essential component of the physician's life and profession? Or is it that ethics is only a formality, and after the ceremony, it is business as usual? One way out of these doubts might be to dwell on the thought of Sandra Gold: "every physician in training should spend a week as a patient" (Gold and Gold 2006, 549). Recounting the narrative of one medical student whose mother died of pancreatic cancer, she quotes:

> *I returned to school and slowly caught up, but I was changed. I returned with the perspective of family. I knew what it was like to have a refrigerator full of medicines, to take drugs only to counter the side effects of other drugs, to be powerless. I learned how much our health can affect those around us and how a care provider must often work with an entire family of hopes and fears, and I came to see, truly and deeply, that the reason for those texts, and those microscopes, are our mothers and wives, our children and neighbors, our colleagues and teachers, our patients (2006, 249).*[10]

This thought has been recently put to practice at the University of New England, where, a thirty-eight-year-old medical student, Kristen Murphy, learned first hand what it means to be dependent on others in one's daily chores. While studying to

---

10. My emphasis.

become a geriatrician, she lived in an elderly nursing home as an eighty-five-year-old stroke patient (Zezima 2009). One might argue that this program is laudable, but not practical, as most of the elective courses that medical students take do not exceed four weeks in duration. Yet, one can argue that something shorter, within the same spirit, might become a universal requirement. Having every medical student work as a nursing assistant for a week would provide a good learning experience for a start. The same idea was introduced in 1991 towards the end of the film *The Doctor* (Haines and Ziskin 1991). After becoming a patient and realizing what it means to be on the other side of the stethoscope, Dr. Maggie requires that his students all wear hospital gowns, eat hospital food, undergo tests, and live the life of an in-patient for a week. After students undergo such experiences, the white coat ceremony would be more meaningful and effective as a curricular event. Students would come to appreciate the elements that constitute what it means to be a doctor and what the white coat really represents. These are encapsulated in the physician-patient relationship.

I have established the importance of the hidden curriculum and the organizational culture in the prevalent paradigm shift that inevitably is taking place in modern medical education. Yet, one cannot deny the prevalence of an important matter for educators to ponder: How can one measure and assess the content, process, product, and outcomes of the hidden curriculum? More will be said about this in chapter four, when the practical implications of clandestine curricula in medical schools will be tackled.

3.1.5. The Informal Curriculum

The informal curriculum is often confused with the hidden curriculum, although they are two different things. The informal curriculum entails the way one sees people treating each other, and the way one sees oneself being treated. Thus, the informal curriculum is part of the social environment of the student. According to Wade Gofton and Glenn Regehr, the informal curriculum "is the process by which a learner's knowledge and skills become situated in the context of daily work. It is not structured but is opportunistic, with appropriate lessons being offered when appropriate learning opportunities arise" (Gofton and Regehr 2006, 20). It takes place in the coffee shop, the elevator, the hallway, the wards, and so forth. In other words, it occurs almost continually in unexpected sites. Pellegrino and Thomasma argue that "the most effective instruments of character formation are the professionals who teach in medical and law schools and seminaries. But they must be able to *demonstrate* that competence and character are inseparable" (1993, 158).[11] Indeed, medical students quickly learn the rules of appropriate and efficient behavior by seeing those with influence behaving one way or another (Hilton 2004). This makes the informal curriculum a fecund ground for effective influences on vulnerable and impressionable students who, directly or indirectly, find themselves emulating those they perceive as role models.

3.1.5.1. Role Models in the Informal and Hidden Curricula

Role models teach by example, motivate, enthuse, and leave a long-lasting imprint on the neophyte physician (Ambrozy et al. 1997; Wright 1996; Wright et al. 1998; Reuler and Nardone 1994). Scott Wright and his colleagues maintain that teaching the psychosocial aspect of medicine is viewed by students as excellent faculty role modeling, noting that "many of the attributes associated with being an excellent role model are related to skills that can be acquired and to modifiable behavior" (1998, 1986), which is quite an Aristotelian perspective to acquiring virtues. Nevertheless, there is no magic recipe that makes one a good role model. Physicians often don't realize that they are role models to students, and negative role models equally play a role in the shaping of the future physician (Mutha et al. 1997). In one prominent university, a third-year medical student, after witnessing an attending physician charging patients without seeing them by asking students to put his name on their charts, reported to his ethics professor that, although he disagrees with this behavior, he sees that it is lucrative and an easy way to make money. When asked whether he would consider doing that in the future, he replied that at times he might feel tempted to do so. This is precisely why good role models should be identified and chosen to spend more time with students. Indeed, some medical schools like the University of Chicago Medical Center, Indiana Academy of Family Physicians, and Baylor College of Medicine have respectively established awards such as the Physician Role Model Award, the Indiana Family Physician of the Year Award, and the Ben and Margaret Love Foundation Bobby Alford Award for Academic Clinical Professionalism. Osler contended that mentoring and teaching were inseparable. He came up with a fresh method in medical education that consisted of teaching by example. He was viewed as a role model, an ideal to be emulated and followed by students and generations to come. Yet, the question arises as to whether a role model has to be a heroic or saintly moral exemplar.

---

11. My emphasis.

In his influential article "Saints and Heroes," James Urmson disputes the traditional threefold classification of moral action in terms of the obligatory, the permitted, and the prohibited (1958). He argues that there is yet another morally significant class of actions: that of the saintly and heroic, that falls outside of the traditional three categories. To illustrate this kind of action, he gives the example of a soldier who throws himself on an exploding hand grenade in order to save the lives of his comrades (1958, 202). According to Urmson, this action falls under acts that are good to do, but not bad not to do. Such supererogatory acts are morally admirable, but are not obligatory, and hence, if one fails to do them, one cannot blamed or held accountable. Should a physician role model be heroic or saintly in the Urmsonian sense? Indeed, the possibility of there being an Urmsonian physician is not farfetched: it is in that sense that one can have a remarkably dedicated, candid, and kind doctor who spends a good portion of her time exercising great communication skills to comfort her patients and is willing to walk the extra mile for them, even to show instances of rising above self-interest and espousing a form of self-effacement.[12] Yet, does that make the physician a good moral exemplar? One can argue that Urmson's example of the soldier sacrificing his life by throwing himself on the grenade to save others is quite un-Aristotelian. Is he not moving away from the mean towards excess? Furthermore, is this all there is to him? A soldier? What about concern for his family, for example? Does he have no obligations other than to his squad? By his colleagues, he is hailed as a hero and a martyr, and it might be the same with his family as well. But that does not mean that, along with feelings of pride, his family does not experience a sense of betrayal for being left behind. The same applies to the physician who delves into excesses. Consider the following case: after an earthquake, an emergency department physician, rotating with the paramedics, goes into a collapsed building to help victims. One of them has his hand trapped under rubble, and the wall above is about to crash down on top of him. He pleads: "Please do not amputate my arm; please don't." The physician/ surgeon acquiesces and instead does her best to save him without amputating, while waiting for firemen to come and help rescue him. This takes much time, and puts the doctor's life in danger as well as the patient's; is this heroic? What about taking in to consideration her five-year-old daughter at home and the family of the victim—as he is their sole breadwinner? It all depends on the angle from which one is looking, but life is not a movie one can observe from whichever angle one wants.

---

12. Pellegrino and Thomasma (1993) spoke of self-effacement as a necessary virtue for physicians. This virtue is not much different from the conventional ethics of medicine that bids physicians to put the good of their patients above their own self-interests.

It is a whole, and the right action must take the whole into consideration; otherwise else "heroic" becomes another word for "excess." Thus, it seems that, at its best, the Urmsonian vision of saints and heroes can be seen as a framework within which to operate. The virtuous physician would be one who strikes a mean between excesses and hence, only in this sense, is an Aristotelian hero. Virtues and ideals can motivate physicians to go the extra mile, but this extra mile often passes through foggy terrain. Treating patients with SARS or swine flu might be seen by many as a duty and not a supererogatory act since society bestows certain privileges on health professionals and expects in return that its sick members be treated. Physicians put themselves at risk while treating patients, and some see this risk as a duty while others see it as a heroic act. Consider Dr. Rieux in Camus' *The Plague*, who commits himself to fighting a highly contagious plague against all odds, and Florence Nightingale, who went the extra mile to tend to patients when others had retired to rest. Indeed, such doctors are hailed as heroes (Hsen and Macer 2004). Looking at the issue differently while acknowledging the existence of saintly and heroic ideals, Childress and Beauchamp argue that many beneficent actions by healthcare practitioners belong somewhere between "weak obligation" and "beyond obligation"—which is a weak form of supererogation—like assisting a visitor lost in the hallways of the hospital (2001, 42). Notwithstanding, as stated by Michael Kottow, "[r]ecurring discussions on supererogation appear to reflect the need to see health services in a light more ample and generous than a contract between health providers and patients" (1990, 124). Thus, is the physician (or ought the physician to be) someone who seeks to promote beneficence (who promotes the good of the patient), a Levite (bound by a clearly stated set of rules), a Samaritan (who seeks to help when she is not obliged to), or an altruist with supererogatory bents? According to Kottow, "common to all descriptions [save the last one] is that they obtain under tolerable cost-benefit conditions, that is, Levitism, Samaritanism and beneficence do not require costs from the agent in any way equivalent, much less in excess of the harm being averted" (2001, 125). He concludes that medicine is a "non-magnanimous service" (2001, 127); it is unfair and dangerous to require physicians to be supererogatory, and it is "better to limit ethical demands on physicians to the feasible and controllable instead of unsettling professional conscience by demanding supererogatory standards that are hard to specify and therefore equally hard to fulfill" (2001, 127). Beauchamp and Childress conclude with an example of the obligation to treat patients with HIV, stating that:

> *. . . proposed policies have been controversial, and professional codes and medical association pronouncements have varied extensively. We*

> *probably cannot resolve such issues without considering the level of risk
> that professionals are expected to assume and setting a threshold beyond
> which the level of risk is so high as to be optional rather than obligatory
> (2001, 43).*

This is why, they add, referring to an article by George Annas (1988), some medical associations require their physicians to exhibit the virtue of courage and to treat HIV patients while others advise them that treatment is an optional matter, and others still stress the virtue of self-effacement and the duty to treat patients. According to the instigators of principlism, such extraordinary persons are often considered role models, and among these role models, the moral hero and saint are the most illustrious (2001, 46). They correctly note that one often learns about virtuous behavior from "persons with a limited repertoire of exceptional virtues, such as exceedingly conscientious health professionals" (2001, 46). They give the example of John Sassall, a doctor who chose to practice medicine in a poverty stricken country in the mid-1960s, and they extract four criteria of moral excellence: the agent 1) has a worthy moral ideal; 2) has a motivational structure in the sense that he is disposed by good character to have good motives and desires; 3) has an exceptional moral character that allows him to perform supererogatory acts; and 4) is a person of integrity (2001, 47). These criteria, according to the authors, "appear to be sufficient conditions of moral excellence" (2001, 47). If one is to argue for virtuous moral exemplars based on this conception, this is not a Sisyphean task. Put in Aristotelian terms, each person should aim at a level as lofty as his potential allows. Some physicians are more prone than others to become moral exemplars, some even moral heroes and saints, but we cannot, nor should we, require all physicians to be like that. This is why to argue for heroism and saintliness might make the task altogether too difficult. Heroes and saints are inspiring, but one cannot demand that a physician be a hero or a saint. One has to choose to become one oneself, which represents an added excellence to be lauded.

Notwithstanding, it is my contention that we can and indeed should require that physicians be at least virtuous. Childress and Beauchamp hold that the person they will "recommend, admire, praise, and hold up as a moral model is the person disposed by character to be generous, caring, compassionate, sympathetic, fair and the like" (2001, 29).[13] Here the importance of character education and the role of virtues becomes apparent (cf. chapter two). When physicians have good character

---

13. Although they do add that character alone is not enough and action must be judged to bring about the wanted results and must abide by the relevant principles and rules (Childress and Beauchamp, 2001, 29).

and are virtuous, it is safe to require or expect them to play the role of good mentors. In his "On Forgetting the Difference Between Right and Wrong," Gilbert Ryle argues that the "notion of moral non-education is familiar enough, but the notion of moral miseducation has a smell of absurdity" (1958, 159). Physicians often profess to know good from bad and right from wrong, yet unfortunately, this is not always reflected in their everyday practice, and as such they cannot be good mentors and role models. Ryle maintains that, just as it appears inconsistent to say that a person knows the difference between good and bad wine or poetry without caring more for one than the other, it is difficult to imagine a person (a physician for our purposes) who claims to know the difference between good and bad action while caring less for it. Thus, there is an interconnection between knowing and caring, between a person (a physician) "knowing that something wrong had been done, but still not disapproving of it or being ashamed of it; of his knowing that something would be the wrong thing for him to do, but still not scrupling to do it" (1985, 152). Thus, the question arises whether such physicians were virtuous to begin with since they did not lack knowledge of right and wrong but lacked that extra something that made them act in the right way. Ryle adds, with a rather Aristotelian twist, that coming to know is also "coming to admire or enjoy" (1985, 154).[14]

Role models not only influence the career choices of medical students, they also leave an imprint on the kind of physicians their students will ultimately become. The informal curriculum is "the overt influence of the hallway conversations, dining room and dormitory talk, comments on rounds, and ways of treating persons on the wards to which students are exposed" (Branch, 1998, 741), and hence, it plays a crucial part in forming the professional identity of the future physician— perhaps, most importantly, a self-image of what kind of professional she will become. The hidden curriculum functions like an invisible hand, and its impact is enormous. As Frederic Hafferty and Ronald Franks assert:

> [m]edical training is not just about the acquisition of new knowledge and
> skills, it is about the acquisition of a physician identity and character.
> Initiates arrive at the gates of medical school with established values.
> They do not, however, leave medical training with those values intact or
> unmodified. More to the point, they are not supposed to exit from the

---

14. Ryle does admit that moral deterioration occurs; yet he argues that what he is denying is that "such deteriorations are to be assimilated to declines in expertness, i.e., to getting rusty" (1958, 150–151).

training process unaltered—at least as far as the culture of medicine is concerned (1994, 865).[15]

In several teaching hospitals, the hidden curriculum suffers from moral erosion. Students often leave the classroom only to see that what they learned in a medical ethics class about patient autonomy is not respected. An example would be when an obstetrics and gynaecology attending physician requests that a pelvic exam be done on a sedated woman who has not consented to the examination. Consequently, the gap between theory and practice widens and is often filled schizophrenically unless one of two things occurs: 1) students have already identified their *phronimos*; or 2) students are armed with moral courage and have the valor to speak up. Thus, in order to reinforce the moral development of students and to ensure that moral erosion is minimized, if not eliminated, a number of activities need to be done to support, enhance, and/or improve role modeling. As role modeling involves a certain approach in ethical training which exposes trainees to particular attitudes, character traits, and behaviors, and, more specifically, to individuals in whom these attitudes and character traits are embodied, various training activities can be envisaged to enhance this aspect specifically. This might include faculty development programs such as conferences and workshops that deal with issues related to areas like virtues in medicine, mentoring, and the hidden curriculum; peer group discussions akin to a "safe space" where peers discuss what they see on the floors, share their concerns about good and bad role models, and learn from both; ethics rounds where the clinical ethicist goes on rounds with the medical teams and they discuss the ethical sides of the issues, when there are any, identifying best practices in medicine, connecting them to role modeling, and using them as teaching moments; and grand rounds in practical ethics, tackling issues related to the hidden curriculum, the importance of being a good role model, and mentoring. This would instill the feeling that the institution takes these matters seriously, and that caring for what it means to be a good physician is part of the culture. And, perhaps most importantly, it would provide exposure to views from the perspectives of the patients, which can be done through ethics consultations, talking with patients, listening to what they have to say, and using these as learning moments.

When asked what it feels like to be old, thirty-three-year-old Mrs. Ramirez replied, "painful and frustrating." She partook in a three-hour training program entitled "Extreme Aging," intended to imitate the weakened capacities linked with old age

---

15. Italics in original.

(Leland 2008). Forty-six-year-old Kim Hansen, who also took the course, emphasized that the toughest part of the experience was having to suffer losing people who filled her life: "I gave up my parents first . . . then it was between my husband and my kids. . . . I got very emotional with that" (Leland 2008). Exercises like this trigger a person's imagination in a way that allows one to come close to what others feel. They allow one to experience Martha Nussbaum's empathy: an "imaginative reconstruction of the experience of the sufferer" (Nussbaum 2001, 327). Ethical thinking has to move a little further into the realm of moral imagination for the student of medicine to ponder what life might be like for the person on the other side of the stethoscope. The same exercise must be done not only with students, but also with attending physicians, who tend to forget what it means to be a patient. A week's stay in the hospital, wearing patients' clothes, eating patients' food, and undergoing tests and other ordeals would remind them of the other side of the equation. Most importantly, what is needed is an organizational culture that supports both ethics teaching and a culture of ethics and professionalism.

One can thus argue that medical education is not something that is simply "offered"; rather it is something that is "acquired," and this acquisition takes place at different levels. It can be direct, like formal education and direct tutoring, and it can simply happen through what I call the "clandestine curricula," as in the hidden or informal curricula. Yet, in addition to the hidden and the informal curricula, there is also the "phantom curriculum" that one cannot afford to overlook.

3.1.6. The Phantom Curriculum

According to Leslie Owen Wilson, the phantom curriculum is defined as the "messages prevalent in and through exposure to any type of media. These components and messages play a major part in the enculturation of students into the predominant metaculture, or in acculturating students into narrower or generational subcultures" (2005). An example would be the increasingly popular TV medical drama. A great number of medical students watch medical dramas like *House MD, Scrubs, Chicago Hope,* or *ER*. According to Jeffrey Spike, "there should be no shame in admitting that sometimes professional scriptwriters can write a better script than a small team of doctors and ethicists working in isolation at a medical school as if it were a cottage industry" (O'Reilly 2009).[16] The medical drama has a specific appeal

---

16. The source of this quotation was a 26 January 2009 article in the journal *American Medical News* entitled

to students of medicine, as is the case with Fox's *House MD*, whose hero, Dr. House, communicates with diseases instead of patients. Dr. House is an acerbic physician who practices most of his doctoring on the whiteboard instead of at the bedside, which, to many of the physicians who teach ethics and belong to the Oslerian tradition, is the first infraction in medical practice. In the pilot episode, a notorious yet memorable conversation takes place between this tragic hero and his assistant which sets the tempo of the episodes to follow:

> Foreman: *Isn't treating patients why we became doctors?*
> House: *No; treating illnesses is why we become doctors. Treating patients is what makes most doctors miserable (House MD,* Pilot, Episode 101).

An essential feature of the series is the bitter and paradoxical character of the protagonist. House is an antisocial drug addict who liberally consumes Vicodin for chronic leg pain and employs bizarre means of diagnosis and treatment. He habitually risks the lives of patients in attempting to save them. This is another questionable type of behavior that is often debated when considering the ends of medicine. His "epiphanies" are paved with what are judged immoral resolutions, and he is often contrasted with his friend, Dr. Wilson, a kind oncologist who is almost everyone's favorite physician. Put plainly, House's hubris is tragic. Still, the massive popularity of the show cannot be dismissed, as ratings indicated an average of fourteen million viewers.[17] However, a study by Johns Hopkins researchers has found that *House MD* was full of ethical breaches and unprofessional misconduct (Czarny, Faden, and Sugarman 2010). The study's authors state that:

> *Dr. House is a brilliant clinician who has little regard for social interactions, human relationships or common courtesies. He is disrespectful and harsh to both his coworkers and his patients and will stop at almost nothing in the pursuit of the correct diagnosis and best possible treatment for his patients. The physicians working under him frequently display a high level of dislike for him but at the same time are always seeking his approval. The viewer frequently gets the feeling that Dr House's actions are ethically problematic but ultimately acceptable given his enviable single-minded pursuit of the appropriate diagnosis and treatment (2010, 206).*

"TV Doctors' Flaws Become Bioethics Teaching Moments" by K. O'Reilly, archived at https://amednews.com/article/20090126/profession/301269975/2/, but inaccessible at the time of publication.

17. The source of this statistic was a 2006 article entitled "Ratings: *House* doles out ratings dandy" by M. Colin at TV.com, last viewed in 2009 at http://www.tv.com/story/7006.html. It is no longer available online and does not appear to have been archived.

Obviously, what is needed is a neo-Flexnerian revolution to redesign the entire medical learning environment. As Gofton and Regeher argue:

> [i]n moving towards the goal of a truly concordant curriculum, it will be important to ensure this is more than a one-time change. To be successful, we will have to design a mechanism to facilitate continual evaluation not only of the formal curriculum, but also of the informal and hidden curricula to ensure that together they transmit a strong message continuing to meet the changing needs of society. In the meantime, we would encourage each individual front line surgical educator to consider and reflect on the significant contribution they are making to the hidden curriculum on a day to day basis (2006, 26).

Watching medical dramas and films that portray physicians as insensitive and opportunistic may have a negative effect, as some medical students might find in this successful physician a role model, but the opposite is also true. Films and medical dramas that instigate empathy may make medical students more considerate, understanding of patients, and more altruistic. According to Roger Dobson, this is the "Don Quixote effect" where "imagination overcomes reality" (2005, 166). Dobson argues that this effect "could be introduced into the medical curriculum to help medical students develop more compassion, kindness, and caring" (2005, 166). Here we witness the fusion of both forms of curricula in the hope of accomplishing one aim—namely, the making of a good physician capable of serving the ends of medicine. In Plato's *Republic,* Socrates contends that "education is not what it is said to be by some, who profess to put knowledge into a soul who does not possess it, as if they could put sight into blind eyes. On the contrary, our own account signifies that the soul of every man does possess the power of learning the truth and the organ to see it with" (1942, 227). Henceforth, education has the job of ensuring that instead of looking in the wrong way, the eyes and minds of students are turned the way they ought to be. Herein lies the role of the medical school when it comes to building the character of the neophyte physician.

3.2. Where Do We Go from Here?

Medical ethics is no longer a new field, as many schools have already incorporated the discipline in their formal medical curricula. However, a problem still lurks on two levels. The first is the physician deep-rooted in a tradition that did not include training in medical ethics and who still thinks of imposed ethics as an intruder, dealing with it and what ensues from it cautiously. To many such physicians and medical teachers, medicine is foremost a science, and medical ethics is something that they *have* to teach, and it ends there. This is particularly the case with physicians who see ethics as a set of rules to be taught and theories to be memorized and/or understood rather than how ethics ought to be seen when it comes to the making of a physician—namely, a way of behaving inseparable from virtues to be internalized. The second problem lies at the level of the clandestine curricula. Here, a paradigm shift has to take place. In certain institutions, it probably has, otherwise we would not have started seeing articles and conferences about the hidden and informal curricula and their impacts. Therefore, just as there was a Flexnerian revolution towards the basic sciences, there needs to be another kind of revolution towards incorporating virtue ethics into institutions that teach medicine so that the formal and the clandestine curricula speak the same language. Even if one were to try to work around a virtue approach like the one elaborated in chapter two, it remains a fact that virtue requires internal and external conditions for it to flourish. If the external environment impedes the development of virtue, it will not prosper, some virtues might even dissipate, and one might see the development of vices (as also explained in chapter two). This is why organizational structure plays a critical role and cannot be underestimated.

In this chapter, I raised the question of whether all students who matriculate into medical school should graduate, an issue that will be addressed in detail in the coming chapter. I also discussed the different kinds of curricula and the roles they play in the making of the neophyte physician. The central issue of this chapter was the role that curricula play in helping students acquire needed character traits that will allow them to *do the right thing even when no one is looking*. Another important question remains: What can one do in order to ensure that, practically speaking, students of medicine will internalize that dictum and that they will not be victims of moral schizophrenia? Put differently, what, on the practical level, should be done to create the virtuous physician? What steps need to be taken in order to ensure that the mentors will model by word and deed the ethical nature of the medical profession in order to produce the student of medicine who will honor the ends of medicine?

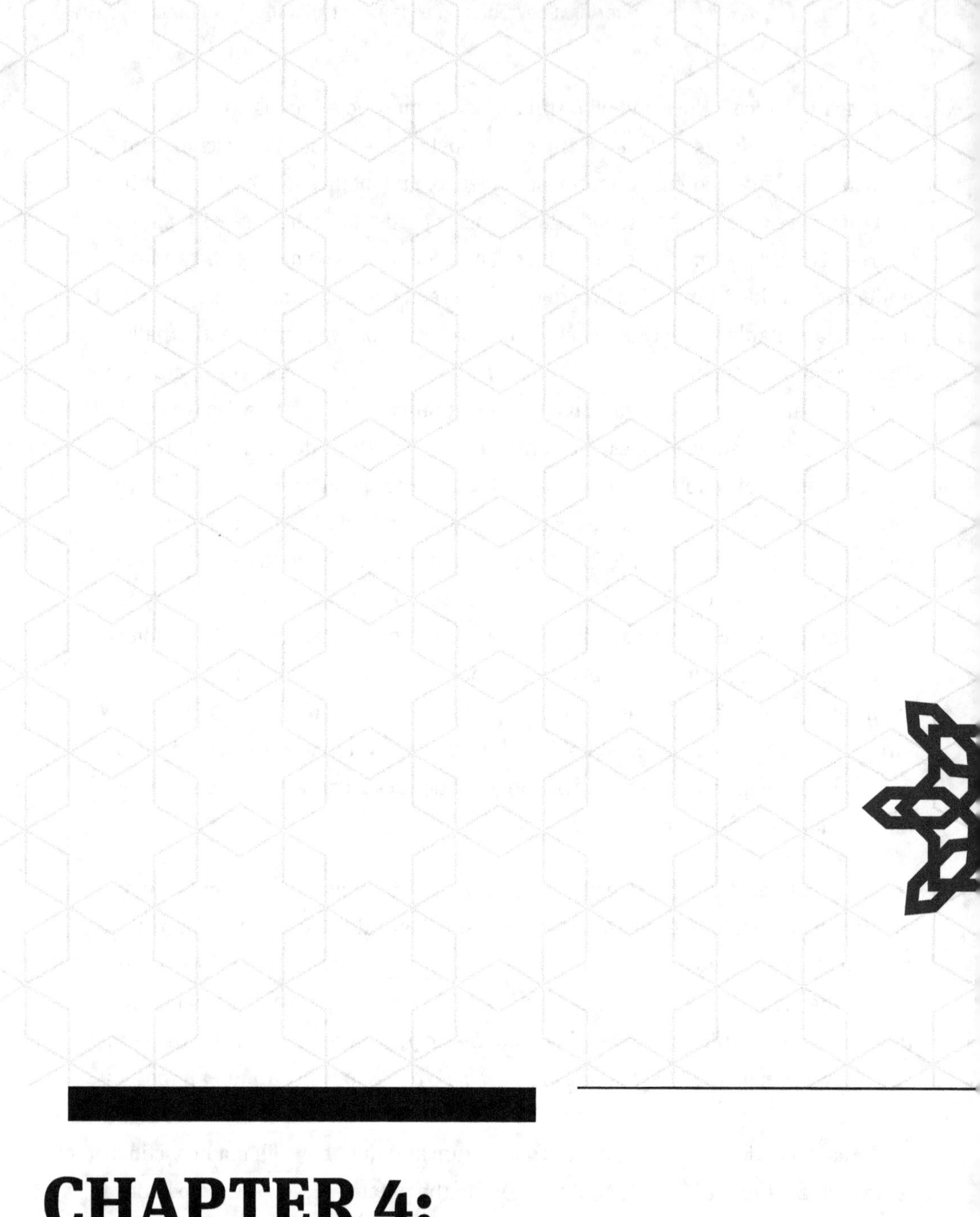

CHAPTER 4:
TOWARDS A POST-FLEXNERIAN REVOLUTION IN MEDICAL EDUCATION

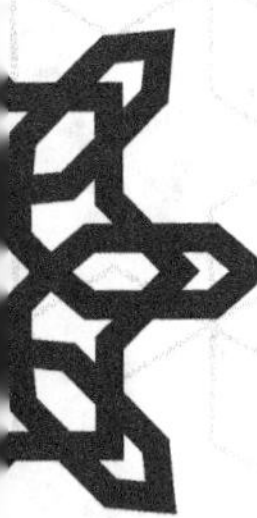

Life is short, the Art is long;
the occasion fleeting; experience fallacious,
and judgment difficult.

—Hippocrates (1939, 29)

"The Palace Thief" is the title story in a collection of four stories by Ethan Canin. It narrates the chronicle of a history teacher at an elite boarding school. The story is a reflection on the vicissitudes of a long affiliation with a spoiled and crooked student, and has been turned into a celebrated movie, *The Emperor's Club*, directed by Michael Hoffman and starring Kevin Kline. Throughout, we see the teacher relentlessly trying to mold the character of the student. "However much we stumble, it is a teacher's burden always to hope that, with learning, a boy's character might be changed. And, so, the destiny of a man," we hear the teacher saying (*The Emperor's Club 2002*). Thus begins the prolonged journey of an attempt at changing the character of a student on the basis of the Aristotelian dictum (quoting Heraclitus), "man's character is his fate" (Canin 2002). The story is an exploration of human relations. At the end of chapter three, I asked: "what steps need to be taken in order to ensure that mentors will model, by word and deed, the ethical nature of the medical profession in order to produce the student of medicine who will honor the ends of medicine?" In this chapter, I try to answer this question by looking at Flexner's Report, an early attempt at changing medical education, and discussing its five key ideas. I argue that there is a need for a post-Flexnerian revolution that will ensure that medical schools will graduate the virtuous physician. As the course of this post-Flexnerian revolution is not without obstacles, some of those are tackled. It will be shown that not everyone who applies to enter medical school should be allowed in, and that even after being admitted, not all who matriculate into medical school should be allowed to graduate and become physicians. Thus, a discussion of admission policies follows. Finally, it will be argued that the virtuous physicians who are already on-board have an important task ahead of them that they need to accomplish in order to create a culture that supports professionalism and the making of the good neophyte physician.

As one enters the Yale School of Medicine, one's eyes are drawn to the façade of the gigantic granite building and the inscription, *School of Human Relations*. When he arrived at Yale in 1917, Dr. Milton Winternitz had a dream, and a few years later, when he became dean, he established the school of medicine, calling it the "School of Human Relations." He visualized it as a haven where social scientists would work in collaboration with biological scientists to study the human being as a whole. Unfortunately, this only lasted a few years (Spiro and Norton 2003). Medical schools continued to encourage a mostly scientific endeavor. After its foundation, the American Medical Association expressed uneasiness about the fact that physicians were poorly trained. Consequently, in 1906, its Council on Medical Education carried out a study of all the medical schools in the nation, only to find out that the entire system was a mess. The only school that was thought to possess the requisites for a good model was the Johns Hopkins Medical School, which was based on the German model of a research university. In 1908, the directors of the Carnegie Foundation for the Advancement of Teaching decided to choose a qualified and knowledgeable researcher, Abraham Flexner, to study the nation's 155 medical schools. His study confirmed the results of the American Medical Association study. The appearance of the Flexner Report (1910) is now considered the most significant event in the history of medical education in the United States and Canada, and it became the driving force that led to modern medical education as we know it. Flexner's Report, as it came to be known, concluded that medicine must be taught and practiced on *a scientific basis*. Herein lay the solution to the problem that medical schools faced; yet, herein also resided the root of the problem that medical schools came to face in later years: they became too narrow-minded in their concentration on research and the basic sciences to the extent that matters of ethics, professionalism, and character became of secondary importance. Nevertheless, Flexner himself was not oblivious to the importance of cultivating the entire physician. Towards the end of the first chapter of his report, he wrote:

> *So far we have spoken explicitly of the fundamental sciences only. They furnish, indeed, the essential instrumental basis of medical education. But the instrumental minimum can hardly serve as the permanent professional minimum. It is even instrumentally inadequate. The practitioner deals with facts of two categories. Chemistry, physics, biology enable him to apprehend one set; he needs a different perceptive and appreciative apparatus to deal with other, more subtle elements. Specific preparation is in this direction much more difficult; one must rely for the requisite insight and empathy on a varied and enlarging cultural experience. Such enlargement of the physician's horizon is otherwise important, for scientific progress has greatly modified his ethical responsibility . . . it goes without saying that this type of doctor is first of all an educated man (1972, 26).*

Ironically, this important and pertinent passage of the Flexner Report is ignored or forgotten by almost all medical schools, as they seem to concentrate less on teaching and much more on research and clinical duties. Indeed, Flexner rightly pointed out that "the enlargement of the doctor's horizon" (1972, 26) is a difficult task, but, along with "insight and empathy" (1972, 26), it is necessary for the physician to be the type of doctor the patient needs: to be precise, an "educated man" (1972, 26). At this point, the following questions arise: What are the practical steps that a medical school can take in order to ensure that its graduating students will have an enlarged horizon and will be the educated persons Flexner referred to? What guarantees that students of medicine will graduate, having met the mission and objectives set by the medical school (referred to in chapter one), and will turn out to be the kind of physicians who will *do the right thing even when no one is looking—* physicians who serve the internal ends of medicine? Put differently, what actions can a medical school take to graduate the virtuous physician? Briefly, the most effective way is the hiring of faculty members who exhibit the requisite virtues in their own behavior. As Aristotle emphasized, the only effective way to teach virtue is through the example of a respected teacher. In the case of medical students and residents, this must be at the bedside as well as in the clinic, with the teaching of bioethics and an emphasis placed on the history of eminent clinicians who have demonstrated the medical virtues in their lives and practices. These can be viewed as ideals to emulate. In addition, one cannot ignore the importance of the supporting power of an institutional environment that encourages and rewards virtuous behavior. In the end, virtuous behavior on the part of physicians will be a reflection of the moral status of the society within which one practices, its educational goals, spiritual integrity, and cultural value system.

4.1. The Flexnerian Revolution

In the US and prior to the Flexner Report, mainstream medical schools were owned by eight or ten faculty members (Beck 2004, 2139; Ludmerer 2010, 193). Institutions were basically operated on a for-profit basis, and the success of the establishment was measured by the amount of profit generated. There were no clear admission requirements, and the courses that were being taught at these schools were sketchy and shallow in nature. The medical degree curriculum consisted of two sixteen-week series of lectures, with the first term being similar to the second. Instruction was basically direct, teacher-centered, and bookish. No laboratory work was done, and students relied basically on memorization. Most importantly, schools were literally "schools," unaffiliated with universities or hospitals (Ludemerer 2010).

Abraham Flexner was a private high school director in Louisville and a firm believer in novel methods of medical teaching. His philosophy of teaching emphasized learning by doing. After being asked by the Carnegie Foundation to study American and Canadian medical schools, he produced a report that posited the following key ideas on medical education (Ludemerer 2010, 194–195):

1) Medicine is basically directed by the laws of general biology.

2) Medical colleges must put in place some admission requirements.

3) The scientific method of thinking was applicable to medicine and henceforth, physicians had to master this method and to apply it in the most cost-effective way.

4) In order to learn, students should spend less time in the amphitheaters listening to lectures and more in laboratories and clinics, thus emphasizing his philosophy of "learning by doing."

5) Research is very important, and physicians should spend a lot of time doing original research. This would also bring thoroughness, enthusiasm, and motivation to teaching.

These ideas were important and played a crucial role in medical schools developing into what they have come to be. Yet, one cannot but reflect on these points and their relation to modern medical schools in an attempt at showing how the views of Flexner should be modified in light of new developments.

4.1.1. Medicine Is Basically Directed by the Laws of General Biology

While it remains true that medicine is basically directed by the laws of general biology, it is a fact that in addition to being biological and anatomical organisms, patients have consciousness and feel and anticipate; they are persons with values and beliefs. It is these characteristics that require a physician to be a physician-healer and not simply a healthcare provider or skilled technician. Hence, medicine should equally be looked at from the perspective of the humanities, for it deals with the patient as a whole. It is in that sense that Pellegrino, in a chapter dedicated to the education of the physician in the humanities, rightly argued that "[m]edicine is the most humane of sciences, the most empiric of arts, and the most scientific of humanities" (1979, 17). This veteran physician who spent around sixty years in clinical practice continued to maintain that the humanities should be pursued "simultaneously with medicine or even later" (1979, 17) as such studies help to "more effectively humanize practice and cultivate the mind of the practitioner" (1979, 17). Interestingly enough, years after publishing his report, Flexner himself felt that medicine had become overwhelmingly scientific. In 1925, he wrote: "Scientific medicine in America—young, vigorous and positivistic—is today sadly deficient in cultural and philosophical background" (1925, 18). As Daniel Sulmasy noted not long ago, healthcare is a practice based on human relationships, and it cannot, and indeed should not, be based on the reductionist view that the ailing person, the patient, is nothing but an assortment of molecular and biochemical reactions to be examined, maneuvered, and manipulated. A patient is a mixture of the biological, psychological, social, and spiritual (Sulmasy 2006). Dealing with the patient as a disease, as an object or tool, dehumanizes the patient and distorts the physician-patient relationship. This is precisely why, at graduation ceremonies or prior to going into the clinical years, medical students partake in the white coat ceremony and take the Hippocratic oath, a mark of their profession, whereby they pledge to honor their commitment to the care of the patient with compassion, integrity, and confidentiality.[1]

4.1.2. Medical Colleges Must Establish New Admission Requirements

This is a very important point that Flexner raised almost a hundred years ago, as a result of which entrance requirements were established. Alas, most entrance standards today do not meet the requirements of the twenty-first century. Premedical (or pre-med) students, as they are now called, have several academic requirements to fulfill before applying to medical school. These requirements entail basically passing a number of courses from across the sciences (including chemistry, biology, and physics) in addition to a language course and electives. Many pre-med students choose their electives solely from the biological sciences, which does little to enhance their exposure to culture and refinement. Prerequisite courses in the history of medicine, medical literature, and bioethics could broaden the horizons of pre-med students and deepen their sensitivities to matters which, although non-scientific, are very important to a future practice as a physician. Talking about the medical humanities, Howard Spiro, a physician from the Yale University School of Medicine

---

1. While oaths may vary among different schools, these are some common tenets that are universally upheld.

argues that "[i]ntroducing these concepts to future physicians should begin before medical school" (Spiro 2006, 997). He continues saying that:

> [s]tudents who identify themselves as "premedical" could have a program less focused on the hard sciences and far more on anthropology, history, and relevant literature. Students who think about the humanities in those impressionable college years should be better able to intertwine real human emotions with their later care of patients (Spiro 2006, 997).

Thus, it becomes clear that medical schools need to rethink their premedical course and entrance requirements in a way that will shape the entire person who will become the medical practitioner of the future.

4.1.3. Learning by Doing

This philosophy currently pervades all medical schools of the twenty-first century. Although students are required to take courses in the basic sciences, they ultimately have to go to the laboratories and learn by the bedside, an approach that came to be known as Oslerian medicine. Unfortunately, bedside medicine has become bedside teaching, and patients often have been turned into teaching tools whose rights are abused for the purposes of teaching. While this might not be true of all patients, it is definitely true of some. It is my contention that using patients in this way undermines the profession of medicine and what it stands for. By "using", I mean any involvement of a patient for teaching purposes where their free, explicit, valid consent for that particular purpose has not been granted beforehand (like the case of the patient who underwent a forceps delivery presented in chapter one). Patients might agree to be teaching "tools," as is generally the case in teaching hospitals; notwithstanding, this needs to emanate from consent, either tacit or explicit, and with this consent ensue a number of duties and obligations that the student of medicine and the attending physician must respect. Any abuse of the status of the patient is an abuse of the social contract that the profession of medicine has made with society.[2] Henceforth, while the philosophy of learning by doing might be right, the way it is applied ought to be revised according to certain policies and procedures that safeguard the profession from serious ethical breaches. Policies and practices

---

2. Society has given physicians social standing, respect, autonomy in practice, and the advantage of self-regulation as well as financial rewards, all based on the prospect that physicians would be proficient, skilled, altruistic, ethical, and would deal with the healthcare needs of patients and of society (Cruess and Cruess 1997, 941–952). This understanding constitutes the quintessence of the social contract.

that do not uphold ethics and that endanger patient well-being (for example, that do not take into consideration the autonomy of the patient by ignoring the importance of informed consent) should be altered. Patients should never be treated as tools to be used as a means to an end; they ought to be considered partners in teaching.

4.1.4. Engaging in Original Research

Modern-day medical schools are known as research universities, and most of them follow the adages "publish or perish" and "patent and prosper." While Flexner hoped that research would flow into teaching and be an added value that would enhance the appeal of the teacher, modern-day medical schools reveal that research takes away time from teaching. It is now common knowledge that medical schools rarely promote teachers for teaching well, for being creative, or even for being compassionate and caring for the sick. The reputation and standing of faculty members rests on the number of NIH grants they get and publications they issue. Physicians who are worried about promotion requirements hardly give enough time to teaching, which they often view as a burden that they bear grudgingly, let alone teaching well, and tend to spend even less time seeing patients. Thus, research has become a double-edged sword. While formerly it was thought that distinction in teaching, research, and clinical skills were the marks of excellence, it has become clear that because of the emphasis on research, teaching and clinical skills have suffered. In addition, the mounting turmoil of the healthcare environment over the last few decades has led to the development of conditions that are unfavorable to medical education, as Flexner himself was aware, and in the US in general as well as in Lebanon, "[c]linical teachers have been under intensifying pressure to increase their clinical production—that is, to generate revenue by providing care for paying patients. As a result, they have less time for teaching" (Cooke et. al. 2006, 1340). This has caused faculty to develop a commercial attitude towards their professional life, and students even hear their teachers speak and worry more about the market and the financial revenues than about curing the sick and relieving suffering (Cooke et al. 2006, 1340). Consequently,

> [W]e arrive at our current predicament: medical students and residents
> are often taught clinical medicine either by faculty who spend very
> limited time seeing patients and honing their clinical skills (and who
> regard the practice of medicine as a secondary activity in their careers)

> *or by teachers who have little familiarity with modern biomedical science*
> *(and who see few, if any, academic rewards in leaving their busy practice*
> *to teach). In either case, many clinical teachers no longer exemplify*
> *Flexner's model of the clinician-investigator (Cooke et. al. 2006, 1340).*

Moreover, some physicians, eager to have their names appear on publications for promotion reasons, forget the rules of authorship and research ethics, and go about it the wrong way. For example, they exploit medical students, who do the work on their behalf, and then end up putting their own names on the research instead of those of the students. Such incidents are not anecdotal but happen quite often. The ends seem to justify the means and as a result, Flexner's educated physician seems to have lost her moral bearings in the process.

Thus, one can conclude that while Flexner did his best to revolutionize medical education and to transform it into a full-fledged education that enhances critical thinking and intellectual skill and vigor, what is lacking in today's post-Flexnerian medical education is a moral dimension that will ensure that the student of medicine will acquire the necessary character traits and skills that will make him a good virtuous physician willing to put the interests of patients before her own.[3]

4.2. Medical Education and the Physician of the Twenty-First Century

One of the most important issues that one has to contemplate before looking at the role of education in the making of the twenty-first-century physician is the true purpose of medical education. Back in 1956, the *British Medical Journal* published an article in which George Pickering said, "The proposition that the purpose of medical education is to turn out properly trained doctors would probably receive general assent. There is, however, dissent about what constitutes a proper training and yet more about what kind of doctor should be trained" (Pickering 1956, 4985). The same still holds true today. In 1800, Dr. John Henry Newman wrote that the aim of a physician's education was to yield "a cultured and highly educated gentleman with, quite secondarily, an adequate knowledge of medicine." (Rao 1961, 1234). When

---

3. Indeed, the medical profession today, more than ever before, faces a dilemma in that it finds itself having to choose between two opposing forces (and thus two separate moral spheres): one which stresses the predominance of the profession's responsibility to the sick and the other the predominance of self-interest and the marketplace. One can argue that it does not make a difference if not all schools require the taking of an oath, for the oath itself is not a guarantee that medical students and physicians will act ethically and be virtuous. My criticism is that there need to be other forms of training (formal, informal, and hidden) that will help nurture character traits that will allow for the making of a good physician. On another note, I am not saying that character *alone* is enough. Virtue ethics will always need the help of rules, for human nature is weak.

asked about the reason they join medical school, many students suggest that one of the main reasons is related to their belief that medicine guarantees a certain decent lifestyle that they would like to achieve. Unfortunately, these are the students who ultimately become physicians, yet, this means joining the medical profession for the wrong reasons, which we see has almost always been the case.[4] Back in 1925, Dr. C. C. Bass argued that:

> *Those who are engaged in other pursuits in life are likely to think, upon superficial consideration, that the purpose of medical education is to provide a gainful occupation for those who enter the medical profession. No such purpose could justify it. In the first place, considering the cost of education, the effort put forth, the arduous duties performed, and the sacrifices made, medicine is anything but a money-making occupation. In the second place, personal gain by capitalizing [on] . . . the suffering and distress of our fellow man does not require the knowledge of the facts that are learned through medical education. In fact, those who are so unscrupulous and so heartless as to do this, succeed through ignorance of, or disregard for, the facts taught by medical education rather than by knowing and applying them (Bass 1925, 13).*

Bass added that medical education "equips the physician with needed knowledge and aids him to render health service to those whom he serves" (Bass 1925, 13). He concluded by saying that "the purpose of medical education is the promotion of health, the happiness, the welfare and longevity of mankind" (Bass 1925, 14).[5] Put simply, the purpose of medical education is to prepare the student of medicine to serve the ends of medicine. Henceforth, if medical education does not meet this goal, then something is wrong and has to be remedied. It is my contention that the medical education of the twenty-first century is no longer meeting its goal of serving the ends of medicine, which is to say healing the patient and restoring his health whenever possible and when not possible, relieving his pain. This is not to say that the learning objectives that meet the ends of medicine are not available. For example, the Association of American Medical Colleges (AAMC) published a report in 1998 in which it stated that:

---

4. Students join for the wrong reasons because they have the external ends of medicine in mind, not its internal ends. Two points are relevant here: 1. The external ends of medicine are not part of its essence; 2. If everyone does something (or if it has been the case for some time by most students), that does not make it right.

5. Although with the development of medical technology, it is no longer longevity alone that matters, but issues pertaining to quality of life as well.

> *The goal of medical education is to produce physicians who are prepared*
> *to serve the fundamental purposes of medicine. To this end, physicians*
> *must possess the attributes that are necessary to meet their individual*
> *and collective responsibilities to society. If medical education is to serve*
> *the goal of medicine, medical educators must develop learning objectives*
> *for medical education programs that reflect an understanding of those*
> *attributes (Anderson et al. 1998, 3).*

The AAMC claim that these attributes include the possession of altruism, knowledge, and skill. Under altruism, they stipulate that before they graduate, medical students should demonstrate the following:

- Knowledge of the theories and principles that govern ethical decision making, and of the major ethical dilemmas in medicine, particularly those that arise at the beginning and end of life and those that arise from the rapid expansion of knowledge of genetics;

- Compassionate treatment of patients, and respect for their privacy and dignity;

- Honesty and integrity in all interactions with patients' families, colleagues, and others with whom physicians must interact in their professional lives;

- An understanding of, and respect for, the roles of other healthcare professionals, and of the need to collaborate with others in caring for individual patients and in promoting the health of defined populations;

- A commitment to advocate at all times for the interests of one's patients over one's own interests;

- An understanding of the threats to medical professionalism posed by the conflicts of interest inherent in various financial and organizational arrangements for the practice of medicine;

- The capacity to recognize and accept limitations in one's knowledge and clinical skills, and a commitment to continuously improve one's knowledge and ability (Anderson et al. 1998, 4–5).

This list was published more than a decade ago, but are these objectives being met? The general dissatisfaction with the ethical traits of physicians testifies to the fact that they are not, and this is so not only in American medical schools, but worldwide. Hence, it has been argued that a "physician's lack of humanity is a general complaint in public surveys. The physician-patient relationship is often viewed by the public as being reduced to a *business relationship*, where the patient feels that she is merely a 'client' and the physician simply a healthcare 'practitioner' instead of 'caregiver' and 'healer'" (Arawi 2010, 23).[6] Recalling an incident that happened while attending a conference in London to discuss the medical humanities, Rafael Campo recounts the story of a medical student inquiring about what the medical humanities are and how he wanted to bring up a definition:

> *knowing intuitively that the way medicine is now taught and practiced is simply* wrong, *that the humane is being supplanted by unfeeling science and uncaring economics—the incalculable distress I feel when I hear an intern refer to her patient as "the breast cancer in room 718," the ephemeral sadness in cutting short a visit before we can delve into my patient's grief at the loss of her husband because I have three others waiting (Campo 2005, 1009).*[7]

Physicians themselves are becoming aware that "the way medicine is now taught and practiced is simply wrong" (Ibid.). Put differently, medical education currently is practiced in such a way that students of medicine are not as attuned to the ends of medicine as they ought to be. Rather, they are more prone to see the external ends of medicine instead of its internal ends, and this leads to a form of moral and professional dissonance. That being said, it is my contention that there is a need for a new post-Flexnerian revolution that will ensure that medical schools will end up graduating the physicians they claim they want to graduate, as professed in their mission statements and the objectives referred to in chapter one. This new revolution will have to be at the levels of the formal, informal, and hidden curricula, and its aim should be the making not only of a physician, but of the "virtuous physician." It will be an education that will transmit knowledge, pass on skills, and instill the values of the profession. Having said that, the first matter of concern is the student matriculating into medical school. Should any student with the right academic record become a physician? Put differently, should all academically qualified students who apply to medical schools be accepted, or should medical schools have certain criteria, other than academic requirements, for accepting new matriculants?[8]

---

6. Italics in original.

7. Italics in original, represented here without italics.

8. Ensuring that appropriate criteria are applied is not an easy task. There will have to be a taskforce dedicated for this. Whatever tools are designed will have to be piloted, tested, and validated. Criteria will have to take into consideration the nature of the medical profession, the internal ends of medicine, and the nature of the physicians one wants to graduate in such a way as to measure the criteria that are essential for the practice of medicine, including screening for character traits consistent with certain personality disorders. Traits that have little consequence for the students' interactions with

4.2.1. Admission Policies

Quantitative criteria, including GPAs and MCAT scores, are the basis of most selection processes used in medical schools. With time, they have gained validity and reliability (Davidson and Lewis 1997, 1153–8). Yet this is not to say that academic criteria are the only requisite measures for entry into medical schools. In the year 2000, *The Lancet* reported the story of a physician by the name of Dr. Michael Swango who was "wanted in Zimbabwe for the murder of five patients and the attempted murder of three other individuals" (McCarthy 2000, 1010). According to McCarthy, Swango poisoned his patients for the "thrill and power" that he felt while watching them as they died. The sad and perhaps regrettable part of the story is that Swango's irresponsible and psychotic behavior dated back to his days in medical school and had continued throughout his residency. As a medical student at Southern Illinois University, he became known for his bizarre behavior and for losing patients under his care. He was inappropriately allowed to graduate and to practice medicine in a morally dubious manner (Steward 1999). The question that arises at this point is this: Should the Swangos of the world be allowed to matriculate into medical school to begin with? And assuming they do matriculate, should they be allowed to continue their studies once their deviancy is discovered? And hence, can the medical school be justified in turning a blind eye to several alarming signs of their immoral or amoral behavior? Swango might be an extreme case, but there have been other cases of less severe infringement. In the same year that *The Lancet* published the Swango story, the *British Medical Journal* published an editorial by a medical student attending the Royal Free and University College London Medical School. The student narrated an episode where a colleague of hers overtly cheated on an examination and was caught on the spot. Although the cheater was asked to stand before a disciplinary committee and was reprimanded, she was nonetheless allowed to graduate (Smith 2000, 398). The editorial condemned the decision of the medical school, describing it as a failure in their social responsibility. As a result, the *British Medical Journal* was inundated with mail, some supporting their opinion and others not. The point is that the issue stirred public opinion as a matter of serious importance and impact, yet, it was not properly dealt with by the medical school itself.

William Osler affirmed that "in the physician or surgeon, no quality takes rank with imperturbability . . . coolness and presence of mind under all circumstances"

---

patients and peers should not be a matter of concern. For example, in a society where homosexuals are not tolerated, homosexuality must not be of any significance as far as admission criteria are concerned. The purpose is not to have a society of *similars* (this might even backfire).

(Osler 1932, 3–4). Such important qualities are often left unmeasured by entrance examinations or other admission tests that students are asked to take prior to matriculation into medical schools. Consequently, the General Professional Education of the Physician and College Preparation for Medicine (GPEP) report made a case for the use of assessment of qualitative variables when medical students are evaluated prior to entering medical school (Muller 1984, 1–208). Qualitative variables are defined as attributes of a person's "character, personality, personal or social history that contribute to success as a medical student and physician" (McGaghie 1990, 145). William McGaghie rightly argues that such variables are important for professional competence and hence should be assessed and evaluated among potential medical students, yet, that is not the case (McGaghie 1990, 145). Some authors have argued that "tests of moral reasoning are inappropriate for use as selection instruments" and contended that it would be more valuable to consider individual differences in "moral orientation" (Bore et al. 2005, 266–275).

In 1980, Rudolph Weingartner suggested ten categories in the list of qualitative variables to screen medical students (Weingartner 1980, 922–927). The list consisted of the following attributes: character and integrity, breadth of knowledge, evidence of leadership, geographic preference, genre, race and religious preferences, work habits and motivation for study, personal tendency toward service, altruism, and personal effectiveness. For example, the American University of Beirut Medical Center relies on the scores of the MCAT and the undergraduate GPA in core premedical courses to decide who gets into medical school and who does not. Yet, it recently introduced a structured and semi-structured system of medical interviews where each applicant meets for around an hour with two interviewers, who ask questions and describe ethical scenarios representing moral dilemmas.[9] The students listen to these scenarios, read by an interviewer, and then are asked to comment on them, focusing on the following: ethics, altruism, teamwork, individual vs. societal rights, as well as respect and autonomy for the individual. Interviewers are asked to rate the responses of the candidate without discussing them amongst themselves. Although inter-rater reliability checks have revealed a high correspondence between the scores of the interviewers, to date these interviews have not played a role in the acceptance of the applicant, although the medical school feels that that should be the case, as character is as important as knowledge. The main hindrance faced is the validity of the interviews in assessing the character of the interviewee. After all, the scientific

---

9. It is important to ensure that those who are conducting the interviews are themselves professional interviewers, good role models, and ethical people. Interviewing is an important function, and more than one or two qualified persons should interview each candidate. Also they should be compensated for performing this essential function.

validity of a one-hour interview is thought to be weak or invalid and has to be further assessed.

Clearly, admission committees ought to incorporate a mechanism through which qualitative variables are assessed prior to admission to medical school, as this has a bearing on the kind of physician the student of medicine will end up being. As much as training in the virtues can help mold the character of a neophyte, one cannot ignore the fact that some students are ethically unfit for medical school. Put differently, some students are not fit to become physicians in terms of character. As stated in chapter two, Aristotle maintained that nothing can form a habit opposed to its nature. He also stated that "it makes no small difference, then, whether we form habits of one kind or of another from our very youth; it makes a very great difference, or rather *all* the difference" (1947, 332).[10] Years later, Pellegrino echoed this in a different way, stating that, "[c]haracter formation cannot be evaded by medical educators. Students enter medical school with their characters partly formed" (Pellegrino 2002b, 383). Thus, faculty members in medical schools not only have the responsibility to help neophyte physicians learn good habits of character, but they also must help them get rid of bad ones. According to Aristotle one is able to become good by unlearning bad habits and learning good ones. The same holds of virtues. If one is habituated to dealing unjustly or high-handedly with patients, one can unlearn this habit by treating the patient justly and modestly over and over again. This requires the help and tutelage of the right professional role model who is willing to patiently and relentlessly observe and guide the student, but this also requires the student to be already someone who has the disposition to become good. It is not an easy task, but it is not an impossible one either. The moral development of the student is a crucial task, and enough time should be allocated to it, starting from matriculation all the way through to graduation. The moral and character development of the student can be assessed by a "student professionalism committee" (explained below) that will develop a checklist and follow the student's moral and character development all through his years of medical training until he acquires levels of excellence of character and practical knowledge (the capacity to see what one ought to do or feel in a certain situation). This will become even more apparent when the student starts to enjoy doing the right thing since the truly virtuous person takes pleasure in his virtuous actions. Thus, some characters are more well suited to go into medical school than others. Unsuitable characters must be sifted out from the start, prior to matriculation. Then, once in medical school,

---

10. Italics in original.

the training in the virtues discussed in chapter two will be more effective and will yield better results. This is where the role of an admission committee comes into play. It should consist not only of physicians, but also have at least one bioethicist, a philosopher and a psychologist. The bioethicist is the person versed in clinical ethics who can help in the framing of ethical scenarios and questions suitable for the clinical setting. The philosopher will also play an important role in assessing the validity of these questions, scenarios, and their internal consistency, and will help in drafting questions in such a way as to frame scenarios that will reveal internal inconsistency within the answers of the applicant. The role of the psychologist cannot be overestimated. Not only should she serve on the committee, but she must also be present during the interviews in order to assess the character and personality of the applicant. Thus, psychological tests should be introduced to assess the psychological reaction of the candidate under pressure and in certain stressful situations; questions should be asked that reveal the presence or absence of certain delicate traits of character such as kindness, altruism, selfishness, and so forth. One can also argue that the candidate's school record from the middle and secondary school years should also accompany his application.[11] The importance of this lies in the fact that the emotional growth and the ambitions of the student can be detected through the comments of their teachers, advisors, and peer reviews. A student who was determined to be developing into an aggressive, selfish person would be a good candidate. Alternatively, a student who was reported to be caring, understanding, and a good listener can be a good applicant. One shortcoming of this proposed course of evaluation could rest of the reliability or unreliability of school reports. Hence for this to be implemented, a revolution has to happen at the level of schools as well. Yet, one can safely argue that, in general, students of medicine ought not to be selected purely on the basis of their intellectual abilities, and that there needs to be some form of assessment of their character traits. There have been several attempts to do that, one being the attempt to assess the emotional quotient (EQ) of the student in addition to his intellectual quotient (IQ) (Borges et al. 2009, 565–572). Emotional intelligence was first defined near the beginning of the 1990s by John Mayer and Peter Salovey as "a type of social intelligence that involves the ability to monitor one's own and others' emotions, to discriminate among them, and to use this information to guide one's thinking and actions" (Mayer and Salovey 1993, 432–442). According to Frank Romanelli et al.:

---

11. Needless to say, there are many cases where letters of recommendation are written in an ad hoc manner and do not truly reflect the character or standing of the applicant. This raises the question: should all professors be allowed to write letters of recommendation? Should any letter of recommendation be considered? What should the relevant criteria be?

> *All health care professions are rooted in a need to establish therapeutic*
> *relationships with patients. Within these relationships, the professional*
> *must respond to both the technical aspects of disease as well as*
> *associated emotional aspects. . . . If this theory holds true and with*
> *various managed care and other environmental constraints being*
> *placed upon practitioners from all health fields, it may become critical*
> *for students in the health professions to have emotional intelligence to*
> *provide high-quality patient care (Romanelli et al. 2006, 5).*

As the physician-patient relationship is at the heart of medicine, being able to interpret or understand and handle emotions is an important skill for prospective medical students and a good guide to thinking and acting. Robert Carrothers et al. (2000, 456–463) were the first researchers to apply this theory to medical school admission processes and to develop a mechanism to measure emotional intelligence for use in the selection of students applying to medical school. The result of their study revealed that: the EI instrument identifies applicants who are oriented toward the social sciences and humanities and who have those qualities of emotional intelligence—maturity, compassion, morality, sociability, and calm disposition—that indicate competency in personal and interpersonal skills (Carrothers et al. 2000, 461).

Notwithstanding, some researchers and scholars still doubt the validity and relevance of the introduction of an assessment of emotional intelligence into medical school entrance examinations. Peggy Wagner, for example, thinks that "such inclusion may be premature" (Wagner 2006, 477). Still, according to a commentary in the *Journal of the American Medical Association*, training in emotional intelligence can assist medical residents and fellows to develop into more sensitive healthcare practitioners vis-à-vis their patients (Grewal and Davidson 2008, 1200–1202). Thus, it is worth investing more time and effort in deciding the role emotional intelligence plays in the physician-patient relationship, and if the correlations are found to be positive, assessing medical school applicants on this basis should be highly recommended.

Although one might argue that what follows is mere speculation, as an applicant to medical school, Swango would most probably not have passed the interviews or the tests suggested by Carrothers et al. If interviewers were careful enough, if psychologists were attuned enough, an alarm would have rung, and such students would not have had the chance to graduate and do the harm they did. Another issue that was raised at the beginning of this section was whether matriculated students should be allowed to graduate no matter what. Several authors have asserted that assessment of readiness for medical education should not be restricted to academic qualification (Puschmann 1966). Rather, character qualifications should also be taken into consideration. Indeed, in the early 1970s, the Association of American Medical Colleges started to introduce changes in the methods of assessing applicants for medical schools. The purpose was to include assessment of character traits in the MCAT; however, the project was soon abandoned (McGaghie 2002, 1085–1090).[12]

4.2.2. Not Everyone Should Graduate

Graduation rates at medical schools have always been very high. For example, at the American University of Beirut Faculty of Medicine, it has always exceeded 96–97%. The remaining 3–4% includes students who fail or withdraw and/or students who decide to pursue an MD-PhD program outside the institution and abroad. No student has been asked to leave the university because of ethical reasons or character issues. Yet, cheating and ethical infractions such as betraying confidentiality, signing informed consent forms on behalf of attending physicians, and participating in dubious research do occur. Papadakis and colleagues have published a number of studies indicating a close correlation between problems with professionalism among undergraduates and residents and subsequent reporting to medical boards (Papadakis et al. 2001, 1100–1106; Papadakis et al. 2004, 244–249; Papadakis et al. 2005, pp. 2673–2682; Papadakis et al., 2008; pp. 869–876). Hence the question: should all students who matriculate be allowed to graduate simply because they meet graduation criteria by successfully completing courses, or should moral requirements play a role? Put differently, should everyone who enters medical school be allowed to become a physician? Pellegrino rightly pointed out that:

> *[t]he prime task of medical schools is to prepare new physicians with the skills and knowledge that would make them safe and competent practitioners after graduation. This in a significant degree implies some conscious shaping of the character of medical students so that they will exhibit, then as students and later as practitioners, those virtues entailed by the idea of a profession (Pellegrino 2002b 384).*

---

12. It is unclear precisely why they let go of the humanities sections (roughly encompassing knowledge of current events, sociology, character traits, and so forth). It is probable that they thought the interview process and essays could offer a better measure of such matters.

It is my contention that medical schools should not educate students only in skill and scientific competence, but as importantly, they should also educate the students in character. A recent study has revealed that the public believes that the majority of physicians are quite skilled in technical expertise, but sometimes lack ethics and interpersonal skills (Arawi 2010, 22–29). This proposed change in graduation requirements implies setting standards below which students of medicine should not fall, and if they do, certain measures ought to be taken to correct this. Henceforth, students who exhibit character traits that do not suit the profession of medicine, students who were admitted to the school of medicine in error and who fail to sufficiently develop the desired virtues of medical professionalism, should not be allowed to stay, even if their grades in medical sciences courses are quite high. These students, it can be argued, might eventually grow into wrong exemplars like the aforementioned Dr. Swango or the Nazi physician, Dr. Josef Mengele. This implies a new change in graduation criteria and a commitment on behalf of the medical school's admission and graduation committees to set new standards. For example, during their four years of medical school, and before they graduate with an MD degree, each student must be closely monitored by an advisor who works with a core committee (let us call this the "student professionalism committee") and evaluates the student's ethical standards two or three times a year. The core committee will consist of the advisor and some members of the medical faculty who are known for their character and honesty and will follow up on the students' development during the year.[13] Students whose ethics and character are found to be dubious or wanting should be asked to leave medical school even if their grades in the curriculum subjects are up to standard.[14] Matriculation should not be a guarantee of graduation as is the case in many medical schools. After all, medical schools will not be asking for anything more than what is already stated in *Harrison's Principles of Internal Medicine*:

> *No greater opportunity, responsibility, or obligation can fall to the lot of a human being than to become a physician. In the care of the suffering, he needs technical skill, scientific knowledge, and human understanding. He who uses these with courage, with humility, and with wisdom will provide a unique service for his fellow man and will build an enduring edifice of character within himself. The physician should ask of his destiny no more than this; he should be content with no less (Harrison et al. 1950, 1).*

---

13. How to assess these character traits and other important ones in faculty members is an issue well worth studying.
14. This will not be easy to do; however, many policies have started out as difficult to endorse, but then became regular policies.

Tinsley Harrison and his colleagues were, in a way, reiterating Hippocrates' claim that the building of character is a lifetime undertaking. They also suggested that the development of character constitutes an important purpose that education has to seek to achieve. In keeping with Aristotle, we sense that the physician who ends up having built an "edifice of character within her" will be happy. Thus, the important role of education in helping shape the character of the neophyte student of medicine to contribute to his growth into the good and happy physician in whom society can place its trust.

4.2.3. The Curriculum and the Professional Physician

Numerous articles have been written recently about the deprofessionalization of medicine (Reed and Evans 1987, 3279–3282; Wynia et al. 1999, 1612–1616; Reynolds 1994, 609–614), a phenomenon denoting the loss of such special characteristics often associated with the traditional physician as commitment to competence, service, and altruism. Consequently, teaching professionalism has recently become an important issue in most medical schools. Indeed, the term "professionalism" has become a mantra reverberating in contemporary medical schools. However, this is not what this section is about, for it is my contention that teaching professionalism in a formal setting will still be prey to the several shortcomings commonly faced by formal courses in bioethics (discussed in chapter three). Rather, what is needed is a "culture of professionalism" that will ensure that medical professionalism and the virtues that come with it will become second nature to new physicians. Thus, another paradigm shift will have to happen and another mini-revolution within medical schools needs to occur, albeit slowly and steadily. Thus, since a culture of professionalism in medical school ought to be established if one wants to graduate the good virtuous physician, the question becomes: how can the medical school curriculum enhance professionalism among future physicians? This will have to be done through the three forms of curricula: the formal, the informal, and the hidden.[15]

---

15. I will not discuss the phantom curriculum here because this is an area over which medical schools do not have direct control.

4.2.4. Medical Curricula, Medical Professionalism, and the Making of the Virtuous Physician

In 2000, Herbert Swick attempted to give a normative definition to the term professionalism. He began by saying that, "the concept of medical professionalism must account for the nature of the medical profession and must be grounded in what physicians actually do and how they act, individually and collectively" (Swick 2000, 614). He thus defined medical professionalism as consisting "of those behaviors by which we—as physicians—demonstrate that we are worthy of the trust bestowed upon us by our patients and the public, because we are working for the patients' and the public's good" (Swick 2000, 614). According to Swick, the term "professionalism" encompasses nine normative behaviors, predominantly humanistic traits such as altruism and honesty, and integrity and compassion.[16] He concludes that "[s]erious negative consequences will ensue if physicians cease to exemplify the behaviors that constitute medical professionalism" (Swick 2000, 616). In 2002, the American College of Physicians published the Charter of Medical Professionalism in *The Lancet* (2002, 520–522). Since the release of the charter, medical schools have grown more aware of it and have started using it to teach medical professionalism, stressing the importance of adhering to a set of professional values appropriate to the profession of medicine. These professional values are very much linked to the virtues discussed in chapter two. Thus, the virtues of medical professionalism were commonly agreed upon to be those expounded by Pellegrino—namely, fidelity to trust, benevolence, compassion, intellectual honesty, courage, and truthfulness (Pellegrino 2002b, 378–384). The question then arises: how should medical schools help their students acquire the virtues of medical professionalism? To begin with, one should concede that medical professionalism and the virtues that come with it are not taught in one single course, and we should not expect that one course (or two or even more) would make students the virtuous professionals we expect them to be. Rather, medical professionalism and its virtues are acquired through the many years of medical training; it is a lifelong project and, as Hippocrates noted, "the Art is long; the occasion fleeting; experience fallacious, and judgement difficult" (Hippocrates 1939, 29). There are times when students will be lured by the negative situations they face

---

16. The nine normative behaviors specified by Swick are: 1) "physicians subordinate their own interests to the interests of others"; 2) "Physicians adhere to high ethical and moral standards"; 3) "Physicians respond to societal needs, and their behaviors reflect a social contract with the communities served"; 4) "Physicians evince core humanistic values, including honesty and integrity, caring and compassion, altruism and empathy, respect for others, and trustworthiness"; 5) "Physicians exercise accountability for themselves and for their colleagues"; 6) "Physicians demonstrate a continuing commitment to excellence"; 7) "Physicians exhibit a commitment to scholarship and to advancing their field"; 8) "Physicians deal with high levels of complexity and uncertainty"; and 9) "Physicians reflect upon their actions and decisions" (Swick 2000, 614–615).

(e.g., conflict of interest, bad role models, and various temptations encountered along the way). Yet, in a healthy and moral medical environment, these erosive forces can be turned into good teaching opportunities that strengthen the virtues instead of weakening them.

There are several publications that help medical professionals teach medical students about medical professionalism. Notwithstanding, it is not the literature that teaches as much as the teachers themselves and the students' experiences. Andrew Brainard and Heather Brislen argue that "the chief barrier to medical professionalism education is unprofessional conduct by medical educators, which is protected by an established hierarchy of academic authority" (Brainard and Brislen 2007, 1010). They wrote their article in order to share their experience as students learning about medical professionalism. The article reveals that in many medical schools in the US, professional virtues are absent and thus teaching medical professionalism and its virtues becomes an exercise in futility. This highlights the importance of creating a culture that supports professionalism and its virtues first among the attending physicians and the educators themselves and then among students. When unprofessional conduct—such as abuse of power, using the patient as a tool, and practicing medicine as a business—is protected by an "established hierarchy of authority" (Brainard and Brislen 2007, 1010), the virtues of professionalism will neither be learned nor will they flourish. Rather, the opposite will take place, and cynicism will increase. At this point, one has to think of one of two things: either only the virtuous and professional physicians ought to be given the task of mentoring and teaching students (which is exigent because these physicians will have to exist and be available in sufficient in numbers to begin with),[17] or one has to start thinking of creating a first generation of physicians who possess these virtues.[18] Both options are difficult. In addition, these physicians will have to be placed in positions of power and equipped with moral courage. They will have to be virtuous possessors of *phronesis* with a strong will to fight a system that has been corrupt for many years.

They will have to work on creating an environment that will reduce student abuse and humiliation, will protect the whistle-blowers by means of a set of policies and procedures, and will create a zero-tolerance policy for physicians who are teachers, yet who exhibit unprofessional behavior. In other words, first on their list of concerns

---

17. Also a mechanism for screening and finding these physicians will have to be put in place, piloted and assessed.

18. The term "mentor" originates with Homer. In Homer's epic, Odysseus went to fight in the Trojan War and entrusted the care of his son, Telemachus, to Mentor. The latter served as Telemachus's teacher and advisor, assisting him to develop the personal, social, and civic skills that helped him gain a good place in society; it was the character of the entire person in question that mattered. Regarding the question of creating a first generation of virtuous physicians, the next question that arises is: how to generate the first generation of virtuous physicians?

will have to be the hidden and informal curricula of medical schools. These virtuous physicians (à la philosopher-kings, but ones who also avail themselves of the advice of other members of the institution) will have a lot on their hands. Among their tasks would be:[19]

1) To develop required courses in bioethics, medical humanities, and the history of medicine to be offered regularly and be given due weight. Integration of bioethics throughout should be considered. Assessment methods used should follow Bloom's taxonomy. Students should also be taught bioethics at the bedside. Ethics rounds can thus be established.

2) To alter the spirit of unhealthy learning approaches among students. Medical training has been described as a journey that enhances competitiveness, individualism, and even deception. These attitudes adopted by students in order to succeed should be avoided, as they stand in exact opposition to the ideals of the physician who should think and act in a spirit of community, collegiality, and teamwork. This disconnect will have to be dealt with early on, and no medical school should tolerate double standards.

3) To arrange the salary structure so that there would be a dedicated body of preclinical and clinical teachers chosen for their teaching excellence and rewarded through bonuses and awards for preserving that excellence. Some faculty members who reveal a lack of aptitude or good character traits should not be permitted to teach, although they could be allowed to continue performing their clinical chores unless their obligations to patient care and ethical skills were in question.

4) To remove bad role models from the core faculty in order to start building a healthy hidden curriculum in terms of professionalism. As Elias Cohen has argued, whatever ill doctors do is often made worse when they are teachers (in Erde 1997, 32). In addition, small details like the decor of the teaching hospital to which the student is exposed need to be carefully considered, As this has a psychological effect on the moral development of the neophyte physician.

5) To be much less tolerant of poor professional performance. It ought not be assumed or taken for granted that everyone who gets into medical school and meets the academic requirements will eventually graduate. Professional and character requirements are as important as academic requirements.

---

19. In order to bridge the gap between theory and practice, an initial "needs survey" is probably required in order to see what students and faculty regard as important for their education.

6) To find faculty "peer-sellers" for bioethics from the various departments and to help create a "hub and spokes model" where a main bioethics resource person (the core hub) would be responsible for sharing ethics knowledge and offering advice, as well as providing support and guidance to designated faculty and staff at the teaching hospital. In turn, there will be "spoke leaders" who will be in charge of supporting others in their departments and programs.[20] Each spoke would consist basically of a program with a designated leader in charge. The leader would, in coordination with the main hub person, who should be a in a position of power and possess *phronesis* (e.g., associate dean for medical education or the director of the bioethics program), designate members who will be working with this leader as mini-spokes, constituting a team. Furthermore, spoke leaders would have their own sub-spokes who would work on developing the program even further. This system would eventually function and spread slowly but steadily as a ripple effect, guaranteeing "integration, sustainability, and accountability" (MacRae, et al. 2005, 256–261).

7) To hold a number of teacher-training sessions at intervals in order to increase the cadre of faculty members who feel comfortable teaching ethics and mentoring students.

8) To work on promotion criteria. Faculty members, mostly as an outcome of the Flexner Report, are rarely promoted for their teaching skills; for being humane, good role models; or for caring for the sick; but rather for the numbers of NIH and foundation grants they get and publications they bring out (regardless of how). The proposed change has to be towards acknowledging the teaching and service faculty, which has a bearing on the making, sustaining, and motivating of the virtuous physician.

9) To formulate policies and procedures that can protect as well as support those trainees who report and seek to change unethical practices.

10) To impose penalties when moral breaches take place. Physicians affiliated with medical institutions who commit serious breaches should not be allowed to continue their affiliations with their institutions. Sanctions should be imposed on a larger scale by the body of medical associations in each country and by the World Medical Association. In the absence of such sanctions, it is the duty of medical schools to call for them.

---

20. An analogous "hub and spokes strategy" has been piloted at the University of Toronto's Joint Centre of Bioethics (MacRae et al. 2005, 256–261).

As mentioned previously, students enter medical school with a measure of idealism. They can become dehumanized or demoralized along the way if they are exposed to wrong role models or if they are abused by the faculty around them, as has been the case in many medical schools.[21] Thus, as good examples of faculty members and actual good ward experiences accumulate and then collide and mix with bad examples of faculty members and bad ward experiences, professionalism and its virtues are either formed or depleted.

4.3. Obstacles Hindering the Post-Flexnerian Revolution

A majority of large medical schools are loaded with institutional impediments that stand in the way of change. As Donald Elliott and his colleagues point out, "[t] heir very structures can be impediments to the horizontal communication and cooperation necessary to effect broad-based innovation" (Elliott et al. 1993, 37). Other challenges include the nature of the curriculum change itself; the degree to which the faculty entrusted to teach the new courses or material are knowledgeable of the subjects they are asked to transmit to the students; the predisposition of the students themselves to be receptive to matters of ethics and whether they are ready for character change (peer pressure being a major obstacle in modern-day society, where anything related to virtues and ethics is seen as a weakness); and disparity between the personal beliefs of faculty members and the values being taught in the new bioethics courses. To this can be added the prevailing time restrictions particularly in an already overloaded curriculum. The problem of territoriality is another serious problem that is often faced when a change is about to take place; when well-established faculty members are not part of the team conducting the change, they may refuse to cooperate.[22] There are also attitudinal obstacles that are hard to deal with. It will be difficult to weed out physicians who, though not virtuous, are well established. As long as these physicians are in the wards, they will continue to be, in one way or another, role models—albeit negative ones—or indirect teachers to at least some neophyte physicians. They will be akin to a virus that could spread and become contagious, and therefore that should be removed from the institution. The problem becomes more pervasive when a physician is highly reputable in terms of skill. The administration should be clear on its priorities. Another serious problem faced is that of the funds that will have to be available to support the changes taking

---

21. See Feudtner et al., "Do Clinical Clerks Suffer Moral Erosion" (1994), referred to in chapters two and three.
22. This can be overcome by slowly involving good people as the spokes of the main programs.

place, from releasing some faculty members and hiring new ones to establishing awards and decorating walls. Finally, and perhaps the most important challenge that arises is that it will indeed be quite difficult to identify the virtuous physician (the philosopher-king) from within the system. One might be identified if already out there, but to be realistic, we might have to wait until such a person graduates from within the institution, which will take much time and great effort.[23] It can happen that this person might parachute in from outside, such as if the school appoints a dean of medicine from outside who happens to possess all the requisite qualities to make the changes.[24] The main point of this argument is that in order to start a revolution—in this case within the medical school—the right revolutionary will have to be found. He or she will have to be a *phronimos*, courageous and determined to make the necessary changes regardless of the obstacles that might be encountered.

4.4. A Return to Virtue Ethics

If one were to actually allow the materialization of all the above, which centers on fostering the desired attributes of a medical professional, the immense challenge lies in minimizing the presence of bad role models among faculty and staff, as well as coming up with a mechanism that will minimize, if not eliminate, the lack of professionalism that is prevalent in most post-Flexnerian medical schools.[25] The question of how to go about doing this is a fundamental one. The most important step in this direction is the alignment of the formal curriculum with the informal (and hidden) curriculum. In other words, all forms of curricula should speak the same language, while the prevailing disconnect will have to be minimized if not altogether eliminated. For this to happen, a revival of virtue theory in the healthcare profession will have to take place. In other words, the professionals involved in the making of what I have been calling the post-Flexnerian revolution will have to be virtuous professionals—virtuous physicians or philosopher-kings. One of the reasons this is necessary as well as possible is the fact that although the theory known as principlism—presented by James Childress and Tom Beauchamp (2001)—has gained wide acceptance for decades, it is now being considered as insufficient for a medical physician to fulfill her professional role. Thus, some argue that the principles are too

---

23. Who is to identify this person and according to what criteria? are pertinent questions.

24. It can also be that this person possesses most of the qualities requisite for making the changes and that he grows in character and *phronesis* as the change takes place through a process of continuous learning and self-maturing.

25. Here again, the importance of the organizational structure appears, but this too will have to be on the list of the virtuous physician. Inevitably, she will have something to start with. Possessing the wisdom that she has, she will know from where to start and how to handle things prudently and diligently.

abstract and removed from the tangibility of clinical experience to the extent that decision-making becomes difficult and too rationalistic, thus holding back empathy and moral imagination (Clouser and Gert 1990, 219–36; Carse 1991, 5–8; Clouser 1995, 219–236). The call for a virtue ethics in professional roles, to use the words of Justin Oakley and Dean Cocking (2001), is in line with the conception of the ends of medicine presented in chapter one which is basically the one proposed by Pellegrino and Thomasma. It is a theory based on the fact of illness (persons become patients when they realize they are ill and dependent), the act of profession (an act of tacit promising to help), and the act of healing (which is basically the telos of medicine). In his *Nichomachean Ethics* (1996), Aristotle talks about the development of virtuous persons and what it means to be a good member of society. In the teaching hospital run by the virtuous philosopher-king, virtuous physicians who will thrive in a good atmosphere and will continue to be trained in the virtues will be nutured. There cannot be a reform of the student without the reform of the faculty, and there can be no reform of the faculty without a reform of the system. It is this reform that will save the medical profession from its downfall and the deprofessionalization to which it has been a prey to for a number of years.

This chapter has dealt with the measures that medical schools can take in order to accomplish the task of graduating physicians who will *do the right thing even when no one is looking*. I have argued that this is done mostly by working with physicians who will serve as role models and mentors in the appropriate institutional culture. For this to happen, a resurgence of virtue theory in medical education is needed. I hope this chapter has made clear that there is a need for a post-Flexnerian revolution that will ensure that medical schools will eventually be graduating the virtuous physician, and that this revolution will ensure that all kinds of curricula speak the same language. It is only then that mentors will model by word and deed the ethical nature of the medical profession, and the schism that separates theory and practice will disappear.

4.5. Conclusion and Suggestions for Further Research

I have argued that medicine is a moral endeavor and the ends of medicine are internal to the profession. As a result, medical schools need to educate students in ethics and the virtues. I have also argued that Aristotle's virtue ethics is a suitable framework for the moral development of medical students during their years of training. Henceforth, virtue ethics ought to play an important role in the formation of the neophyte physician who will *do the right thing even when no one is looking*.

Students become physicians, wear the coat, and feel empowered. In Plato's *Republic* (1942, 43–44), Gyges misuses the power of the ring he found. He uses it to do things that are morally objectionable. In our new medical school following the model of the post-Flexnerian revolution, one might argue that there is a need to guard our virtuous philosopher-king or queen from abusing the powers that they have for purposes other than those for which they were initially given to them. But is there really a problem there? Since we have posited from the beginning that the virtuous physician is a person possessing the requisite virtues and is constantly being trained in them (like Aristotle's athlete), that he or she also has the crowning virtue of *phronesis*, then one can safely argue that the character of this physician- philosopher-king or queen will be kept from abusing or misusing whatever power they may have and that they will continue to *do the right thing even when no one is looking*. That being said, one can also argue that this physician-philosopher-king or queen will be the role model *par excellence*. Henceforth, they can be entrusted the mission of educating future physicians to be the sort of physicians who will *do the right thing even when no one is looking*. They will lead the medical school with a faculty that will help students internalize the virtues of medical professionalism in such a way that they will graduate from the school without having fallen prey to the moral schizophrenia referred to in chapter one, and without succumbing to cynicism and losing sight of what the profession of medicine actually is. For this to happen, students will have to be educated in virtues and not simply follow rules and act out of fear of punishment. They will have to develop a reverence for the profession of medicine and its ends, not a simple adherence to rules and fear of sanctions. In other words, the virtuous philosopher-king or queen can be entrusted to run an institution that will produce the virtuous medical professional. The virtuous student professionals will possess the virtues internal to the practice of medicine. They will, in turn and with time, practice, and emulation, develop their *phronesis*, "medicine's indispensible virtue" (Pellegrino and Thomasma 1993, 84) and will do *the right thing even when no one is looking*.

GLOSSARY

akrasia	weakness of will
akrates	lack of self-control
ceteris paribus	holding other things constant; all things being equal
eudaimonia	happiness, human flourishing, the highest good towards which people aim
ex-nihilo	out of nothing
JAMA	*Journal of the American Medical Association*
Kalon	the ideal good; what is noble and morally beautiful
Mean and all	A term used by Aristotle to mean "any other thing"
NIH	National Institutes of Health
phronimos	a wise resource
phronesis	practical wisdom
praxis	accepted practice or custom
telos	ultimate object or aim

BIBLIOGRAPHY

Abrous, D. N., M. Koehl, and M. Le Moal, M. 2005. "Adult Neurogenesis: From Precursors to Network and Physiology." *Physiology Review* 85, no. 2 (April): 523–569. DOI: 10.1152/physrev.00055.2003

ACP-ASIM Foundation, ABIM Foundation, and European Federation of Internal Medicine. 2002. "Medical Professionalism in the New Millennium: A Physicians' Charter." *The Lancet* 359, no. 9305 (Feb.): 520–522. DOI: https://doi.org/10.1016/S0140-6736(02)07684-5.

Anderson, M. B. et al. 1998. "Report I: Learning Objectives for Medical Student Education Guidelines for Medical Schools". Edited by A. Bradford. Washington DC: Association of American Medical Colleges. Available at: https://www.aamc.org/download/492708/data/learningobjectivesformedicalstudenteducation.pdf.

Albanese, M. A., M. H. Snow, S. E. Skochelak, K. N. Huggett, and P. M. Farrell. 2003. "Assessing Personal Qualities in Medical School Admissions." *Academic Medicine* 78, no. 3 (March): 313–321.

Ambrozy, D., D. M. Irby, J. L. Bowen, J. H. Burack, J. D. Carline, and F. T. Stritter. 1997. "Role Models' Perceptions of Themselves and their Influence on Students' Specialty Choices." *Academic Medicine* 72, no. 12 (Dec.): 1119–1121.

Annas, G. 1988. "Legal risks and responsibilities of physicians in the AIDS epidemic." *The Hastings Center Report* 18, no. 2: 26–32.

Anscombe, G. E. M. 1958. "Modern Moral Philosophy." *Philosophy* 33, no. 125 (Jan.): 1–19. DOI: 10.1017/S0031819100037943.

Arawi, T. 2010. "The Lebanese Physician: A Public's Viewpoint." *Developing World Bioethics* 10, no. 1 (April): 22–29. DOI: 10.1111/j.1471-8847.2009.00258.x.

Aristotle. 1947. *Nicomachean Ethics*. Translated by W. D. Ross. In *Introduction to Aristotle*. Edited by Richard McKeon. New York: The Modern Library.

Arnold P. Gold Foundation. 2013. " What do medical students hope to remember about their White Coat Ceremonies?" Arnold P. Gold Foundation. Available at: http://www.gold- foundation.org/what-do-medical-students-hope-to-remember-about-their-white-coat-ceremony/.

Arras, J. D. 1990. "AIDS and Reproductive Decisions: Having Children in Fear and Trembling." *The Milbank Quarterly* 68, no. 3: 353–382. DOI: 10.2307/3350110.

Atasoylu, A., S. Wright, B. Beasley, J. Cofrancesco, D. Macpherson, T. Partridge, P. Thomas, and E. Bass. 2003. "Promotion Criteria for Clinician-educators." *Journal of General Internal Medicine* 18, no. 9 (Sept.): 711–716. DOI:10.1046/j.1525-1497.2003.10425.x.

Athanassoulis, N. 2006. "Virtue Ethics." *The Internet Encyclopedia of Philosophy*. ISSN 2161-0002. https://www.iep.utm.edu/v/virtue.htm, last viewed 21 February 2019.

Baier, A. 1986. "Trust and Antitrust." *Ethics* 96, no. 2 (Jan.): 231–260.

Basco, W. T., G. E. Gilbert, A. W. Chessman, and A. V. Blue. 2000. "The Ability of a Medical School Admission Process to Predict Clinical Performance and Patients' Satisfaction." *Academic Medicine* 75, no. 7 (July): 743–747.

Bass, C. C. 1925. "The Purpose of Medical Education." *Southern Medical Journal* 18, no. 1: 12–14.

Bazrafkan, L. S., N. Shokrpour, and S. Z. Tabeie. 2008. "A Survey of Patients' Complaints Against Physicians in a Five Year Period in Fars Province: Implication for Medical Education." *Journal of Medical Education* 12, nos. 1 and 2: 23–28.

Beasley, B., and W. Wright. 2003. "Looking Forward to Promotion: Characteristics of Participants in the Prospective Study of Promotion in Academia." *Journal of General Internal Medicine* 18, no. 9 (Sept.): 705–710.

Beauchamp, G. A. 1982. "Curriculum Theory: Meaning, Development, and Use." *Theory into Practice* 21, no. 1: 23–27. DOI: 10.1080/00405848209542976.

Beauchamp, T. L. and J. F. Childress. 1994. *Principles of Biomedical Ethics,* 4th ed. Oxford: Oxford University Press.

Beck, A. 2004. "The Flexner Report and the Standardization of American Medical Education." *Journal of the American Medical Association* 291, no. 17: 2139–2140. DOI: 10.1001/jama.291.17.2139.

Boon, K., and J. Turner. 2004. "Ethical and Professional Conduct of Medical Students: Review of Current Assessment Measures and Controversies." *Journal of Medical Ethics* 30, no. 2 (April): 221–226. DOI: 10.1136/jme.2002.002618.

Bore, M., D. Munro, I. Kerridge, and D. Powis. 2005. "Selection of Medical Students According to their Moral Orientation." *Medical Education* 39, no. 3 (March): 266–275. DOI: 10.1111/j.1365-2929.2005.02088.x.

Borges, N. J., T. D. Stratton, P. J. Wagner, and C. L. Elam. 2009. "Emotional Intelligence and Medical Specialty Choice: Findings from Three Empirical Studies." *Medical Education* 43, no. 6 (June): 565–572. DOI: 10.1111/j.1365-2923.2009.03371.x.

Boyd, K. M., ed. 1987. *Report of a Working Party on the Teaching of Medical Ethics.* London: Institute of Medical Ethics.

Brainard, A. H., and H. C. Brislen. 2007. "Learning Professionalism: A View from the Trenches." *Academic Medicine* 82, no. 11: 1010–1014. DOI: 10.1097/01.ACM.0000285343.95826.94.

Branch, W. T., Jr. 1998. "Deconstructing the White Coat." *Annals of Internal Medicine* 129, no. 9: 740–742. DOI: 10.7326/0003-4819-129-9-199811010-00012.
———. 2000. "Supporting the Moral Development of Medical Students." *Journal of General Internal Medicine* 15, no. 7: 503–508. DOI: 10.1046/j.1525-1497.2000.06298.x.

Branch, W. T., Jr., J. P. Hafler, and R. J. Pels. 1998. "Medical Students Development of Empathic Understanding of Their Patients." *Academic Medicine* 73, no. 4: 361–362.

Branch, W. T., Jr., R. J. Pels, G. Harper, D. Calkins, L. Forrow, F. Mandell, et al. 1995. "A New Educational Approach for Supporting the Professional Development of Third-year Medical Students." *Journal of General Internal Medicine* 10, no. 12 (Dec.): 691–694.

Brody, H. 1992. *The Healer's Power.* New Haven and London: Yale University Press.

Callahan, Daniel. 1996. "The Goals of Medicine, Setting New Priorities," *Hastings Center Report,* Special Supplement, November–December 1996.

Calman, K. 1994. "The Profession of Medicine." *British Medical Journal* 309, no. 6962 (Oct.): 1140–1143.

Campo, R. 2005. "A Piece of my Mind. 'The Medical Humanities,' for Lack of a Better Term." *Journal of American Medical Association* 294, no. 9 (Sept.): 1009–1011. DOI: 10.1001/jama.294.9.1009.

Canin, E. 2002. *The Palace Thief: Stories*. New York: Picador.

Carroll, L., F. M. Sullivan, and M. Colledge. 1998. "Good Health Care: Patient and Professional Perspectives." *The British Journal of General Practice* 48, no. 433 (Aug.): 1507–1508.

Carrothers, R. M., W. G. Stanford, and T. J. Gallagher. 2000. "Measuring Emotional Intelligence of Medical School Applicants." *Academic Medicine* 75, no. 5: 456–463.

Carse, A. 1991. "The 'Voice of Care': Implications for Bioethical Education." *Journal of Medicine and Philosophy* 16 (Feb.): 5–28.

Catholic News Agency. 2008. "Pope reaffirms Church's stance against euthanasia." http://www.catholicnewsagency.com/news/pope_reaffirms_churchs_stance_against_ euthanasia, last viewed 23 November 2011.

Childress, J., and T. Beauchamp. 2001. *Principles of Biomedical Ethics*. New York: Oxford University Press.

Clouser, K. D. 1995. "Common Morality as an Alternative to Principlism." *Kennedy Institute of Ethics Journal* 5, no. 3: 219–236.

Clouser, K. D., and B. Gert. 1990. "A Critique of Principlism." *Journal of Medicine and Philosophy* 15, no. 2 (Apr.): 219–236.

Cohen, J. J. 2002. "Our Compact with Tomorrow's Doctors." *Academic Medicine* 77, no. 6 (June): 475–480.

Colin, M. 2006. "Ratings: *House* doles out ratings candy." TV.com, accessed 12 March 2009, http://www.tv.com/story/7006 (site discontinued).

Conrad, P., and K. Barker. 2010. "The Social Construction of Illness: Key Insights and Policy Implications." *Journal of Health and Social Behavior* 51, Suppl: S67–S79. DOI: 10.1177/0022146510383495.

Cooke, M., D. M. Irby, W. Sullivan, and K. Ludmere. 2006. "American Medical Education 100 Years after the Flexner Report." *New England Journal of Medicine* 355, no. 13 (Sep. 28): 1339–1344. DOI: 10.1056/NEJMra055445.

Coulehan, J., and P. Williams. 2001. "Vanquishing Virtue: The Impact of Medical Education." *Academic Medicine* 76, no. 6 (June): 598–605.

Cribb, A., and S. Bignold. 1999. "Towards the Reflexive Medical School: The Hidden Curriculum and Medical Education Research." *Studies in Higher Education* 24, no. 2 (June): 195–209. DOI: 10.1080/03075079912331379888.

Cruess, R. L., and S. R. Cruess. 1997. "Teaching Medicine as a Profession in the Service of Healing." *Academic Medicine* 72, no. 11 (Nov.): 941–952.

Czarny, M. J., R. R. Faden, and J. Sugarman. 2010. "Bioethics and Professionalism in Popular Television Medical Dramas." *Journal of Medical Ethics* 36, no. 4 (Apr.): 203– 206.

Davidson, R. C., E. L. Lewis. 1997. "Affirmative Action and Other Special Consideration Admissions at the University of California, Davis, School of Medicine." *Journal of the American Medical Association* 278, no. 14 (Oct. 8): 1153–1158.

Davis, A. K., N. B. Kahn, S. A. Wartmann, M. Wilson, and R. Kahn. 2001. "Lessons from the Interdisciplinary Generalist Curriculum Project." *Academic Medicine* 76, no. 4 Suppl: S1– S157.

Dobson, R. 2005. "Medical Students Should Watch Films that Inspire Compassion." *British Medical Journal* 330, no. 7484 (Jan. 22): 166.

Education Committee of the General Medical Council. 1993. *Tomorrow's Doctors*. London: General Medical Council.

Elliott, D., M. L. Hirsch, and M. Puro. 1993. "Overcoming Institutional Barriers to Broad-Based Curricular Change." *Innovative Higher Education* 18, no. 1: 37–46.

The Emperor's Club. 2002. Directed by Michael Hoffman. Written by Ethan Canin (short story "The Palace Thief") and Neil Tolkin (screenplay). Beacon Communications, Universal Pictures. 22 November 2002. DVD. 109 min.

Erde, E. L. 1997. "The Inadequacy of Role Models for Educating Medical Students in Ethics with some Reflections on Virtue Theory." *Theoretical Medicine* 18, no. 1–2: 31–45.

American University of Beirut Faculty of Medicine and Medical Center. 2013. *Faculty of Medicine and Medical Center Catalogue*. Beirut: American University of Beirut. http://www.aub.edu.lb/registrar/Documents/catalogue/graduate13-14/fm-aubmc.pdf, last viewed 3 December 2013.

Feudtner, C., D. A. Christakis, N. A. Christakis. 1994. "Do Clinical Clerks Suffer Ethical Erosion? Students' Perceptions of their Ethical Environment and Personal Development." *Academic Medicine* 69, no. 8 (Aug.): 670–679.

Flexner, A. 1910. Reprod. 1972. "Medical Education in the United States and Canada. A Report to the Carnegie Foundation for the Advancement of Teaching." Bulletin No. 4. New York: Arno Press.
———. 1925. Medicine: *A Comparative Study*. New York: MacMillan.

Foot, P. 2011. "Virtues and Vices." In *Vice and Virtue in Everyday Life*, edited by C. H. Sommers and F. Sommers, 320–335. Boston: Wadsworth.

Fox, E., R. M. Arnold, B. Brody. 2000. "Medical Ethics Education: Past, Present, and Future." *Academic Medicine* 70, no. 9 (Sep.): 761–769.

Gardiner, P. 2003. "A Virtue Ethics Approach to Moral Dilemmas in Medicine." *Journal of Medical Ethics* 29, no. 5: 297–302. DOI:10.1136/jme.29.5.297.

Gaylin, W., L. R. Kass, E. D. Pellegrino, M. Siegler. 1988. "Doctors Must Not Kill." *Journal of the American Medical Association* 259, no. 14 (April 8): 2139–2140. DOI: 10.1001/jama.1988.03720140059034.

General Medical Council. 1998. *Good Medical Practice*. London: General Medical Council.

Gillon, R. 1987. "Medical Ethics Education." *Journal of Medical Ethics* 13, no. 3: 115–116.
———. 2000. "White Coat Ceremonies for New Medical Students." *Journal of Medical Ethics* 26, no. 2 (Apr.): 83–84. DOI: 10.1136/jme.26.2.83.

Gofton, W., and G. Regehr. 2006. "What We Don't Know We Are Teaching: Unveiling the Hidden Curriculum." *Clinical Orthopaedics and Related Research* 449: 20–27.

Gold, A., S. Gold. 2006. "Humanism in Medicine from the Perspective of the Arnold Gold Foundation: Challenges to Maintaining the Care in Health Care." *Journal of Child Neurology* 21, no. 6 (June): 546–549.

Golden, R. 1999. "William Osler at 150: An Overview of a Life." *Journal of the American Medical Association* 282, no.23 (Dec. 15): 2252–2258.

Grewal, D., H. A. Davidson. 2008. "Emotional Intelligence and Graduate Medical Education." *Journal of the American Medical Association* 300, no. 10 (Sep. 10): 1200–1202. doi: 10.1001/jama.300.10.1200.

Hafferty, F. 1998. "Beyond Curriculum Reform: Confronting Medicine's Hidden Curriculum." *Academic Medicine* 73, no. 4 (Jan.): 403–407.

Hafferty, F. W., and R. Franks. 1994. "The Hidden Curriculum, Ethics Teaching, and the Structure of Medical Education." *Academic Medicine* 69, no. 11 (Nov.): 861–871.

Haines, R., L. Ziskin. 1991. *The Doctor*. Burbank, CA: Touchstone.

Harrison, T. R., P. B. Beeson, G. W. Thorn, W. H. Resnik, and M. M. Wintrobe. 1950. "Approach to the Patient. Introduction." In *Principles of Internal Medicine*, edited by T. R. Harrison, P. B. Beeson, G. W. Thorn, W. H. Resnik, and M. M. Wintrobe, 1–5. Philadelphia and Toronto: Blakiston.

Hilton, S. 2004. "Medical Professionalism: How Can We Encourage It in Our Students?" *The Clinical Teacher* 1, no. 2 (Nov.): 69–73. DOI: 10.1111/j.1743-498X.2004.00032.x.

Hippocrates. 1939. *The Genuine Work of Hippocrates*. Translated from the Greek by Francis Adams. Baltimore, MD: Williams & Wilkins.

Hoffman, M. 2000. *Empathy and Moral Development: Implications for Caring and Justice*. Cambridge: Cambridge University Press.

Hojat, M., M. J. Vergare, K. Maxwell, G. C. Brainard, S. K. Herrine, G. A. Isenberg, J. J. Velosky, and J. S. Gonnella. 2009. "The Devil Is in the Third Year: A Longitudinal Study of Erosion of Empathy in Medical School." *Academic Medicine* 84, no. 9: 1182–1191. DOI:10.1097/ACM.0b013e3181b17e55.

House, M.D. 2005–2009. (TV series). Written by D. Shore. Los Angeles: Fox Broadcasting Corporation, Universal Studios.

Hsin, D. H., and D. R. Macer. 2004. "Heroes of SARS: Professional Roles and Ethics of Health Care Workers." *Journal of Infection* 49, no. 3 (Oct.): 210–215.

Hursthouse, R. 1991. "Virtue Theory and Abortion." *Philosophy and Public Affairs* 20, no. 3 (Summer): 223–246.
———. 1995. "Applying Virtue Ethics." *In Virtues and Reasons. Philippa Foot and Moral Theory: Essays in Honour of Philippa Foot*, edited by R. Hursthouse, G. Lawrence, and W. Quinn., 56–75. Oxford: Oxford University Press.
———. 1999. *On Virtue Ethics*. Oxford: Oxford University Press.

Institute of Medical Ethics. 1987. *The Pond Report. Report of a Working Party on the Teaching of Medical Ethics*. London: IME Publications.

Jackson, P. 1968. *Life in Classrooms*. New York: Rinehart & Winston.

John Paul II. 1998. "No Authority Can Justify Euthanasia." *L'Osservatore Romano* (weekly edition in English), 25 November 7.

Johns Hopkins University School of Medicine. n.d. *Medical Student Mission Statement and Education Program Objectives*. http://www.hopkinsmedicine.org/som/mission.html.

Jones, A. H. 1999. "Narrative in Medical Ethics." *British Medical Journal* 318, no. 7178 (Jan. 23): 253–256. DOI: 10.1136/bmj.318.7178.253.

Jonsen, A. R. 2000. *A Short History of Medical Ethics*. New York: Oxford University Press.

Joos, S. K., D. H. Hickam, G. H. Gordon, and L. H. Baker. 1996. "Effects of a Physician Communication Intervention on Patient Care Outcomes." *Journal of General Internal Medicine*, vol. 11, no. 3 (March): 147–155.

Jotterand, F. 2003. "Medicine as a Moral Practice: Reconsidering the Role of Moral Agency in the Patient-Physician Relationship." *The Internet Journal of Law, Healthcare and Ethics* 1, no. 2: 1–9.

Kass, L. R. [1975] 1981. "Regarding the End of Medicine and the Pursuit of Health." *The Public Interest* 40: 11–42. Reprinted in *Concepts of Health and Disease*, edited by A. L. Kaplan, H. T. Engelhardt, Jr., and J. McCartney, 3–30. Reading, MA: Addison-Wesley.

Kassirer, J. P. 1993. "Doctor Discontent." *New England Journal of Medicine* 339, no. 21 (Nov. 19): 1543–1545. DOI: 10.1056/NEJM199811193392109.

Katz, J. 1951. "The Functions of a Profession: Social Status of Medicine and Education." *The Phi Delta Kappan* 32, no. 9 (May): 398–400.

Kenagy, J. W., M. B. Donald, and F. S. Miles. 1999. "Service Quality in Health Care." *Journal of the American Medical Association* 281, no. 7 (Feb. 17): 661–665.

Kenny, N. P., K. V. Mann, and H. Macleod. 2003. "Role Modeling in Physicians' Professional Formation: Reconsidering an Essential but Untapped Educational Strategy." *Academic Medicine* 78, no. 12 (Dec.): 1203–1210.

Kern, D. E., P. A. Thomas, D. M. Howard, and E. B. Bass. 1998. *Curriculum Development for Medical Education. A Six-Step Approach*. Baltimore/London: Johns Hopkins University Press.

Kohlberg, L. 1984. *Essays on Moral Development: The Nature and Validity of Moral Stages*. San Francisco: Harper and Row.

Kottow, M. H. 1990. "Against the Magnanimous in Medical Ethics." *Journal of Medical Ethics* 16, no. 3 (September): 124–128.

Kuhn, T. 1996. *The Structure of Scientific Revolutions*. Chicago: Chicago University Press.

Lasnover, A. 1982. "Cheating Beyond Medical School." *The Western Journal of Medicine* 137, no. 1: 77.

Laurance, J. 2000. "A Medical Student Who Cheated in Her Final Exam Has Been Allowed to Qualify as a Doctor, Despite Being Caught Red-Handed." *The Independent*, 11 August. http://www.independent.co.uk/life-style/health-and-families/health-news/medical-student-who-cheated-in-exam-allowed-to-qualify-as-doctor-710598.html.

Leland, J. 2008. "Simulating Age 85, With Lessons on Offering Care." *The New York Times*, August 3. http://www.nytimes.com/2008/08/03/us/03aging.html.

Lind, G. 2000. "Moral Regression in Medical Students and Their Learning Environment." *Revista Brasileira de Educacao Médica* 24, no. 3: 24–33.

Louden, R. 1984. "On Some Vices of Virtue Ethics." *American Philosophical Quarterly* 21, no. 3: 227–236.

Ludemerer, K. M. 2010. "Understanding the Flexner Report." *Academic Medicine* 85, no. 2 (Feb.): 193–196. doi: 10.1097/ACM.0b013e3181c8f1e7.

MacIntyre, A. 1984. *After Virtue: A Study in Moral Theory*. 2nd ed. Notre Dame: University of Notre Dame Press.
———. 1999. "How to Seem Virtuous Without Actually Being So." In *Education in Morality*, edited by J. M. Halstead and T. H. McLaughlin, 118–131. London/New York: Routledge.

MacRae, S., P. Chidwick, S. Berry, B. Secker, P. Hébert, R. Zlotnik Shaul, K. Faith, and P. A. Singer. 2005. "Clinical Bioethics Integration, Sustainability, and Accountability: The Hub and Spokes Strategy." *Journal of Medical Ethics* 31, no. 5: 256–261.

Maheux, B., C. Beaudoin, L. C. L. Berkson, J. Des Marchais, and P. Jean. 2000. "Medical Faculty as Humanistic Physicians and Teachers: The Perceptions of Students at Innovative and Traditional Medical Schools." *Medical Education* 34: 630–634.

Mansfield, F. 1991. "Supervised Role-Play in the Teaching of the Process of Consultation." *Medical Education* 25, no. 6: 485–490.

Martin, J. R. 1994. "What Should We Do with a Hidden Curriculum When We Find One?" In *Changing the Educational Landscape: Philosophy, Women, and the Curriculum*, 154–169. New York: Routledge.

Mayer, J. D., and P. Salovey. 1993. "The Intelligence of Emotional Intelligence." *Intelligence* 17, no. 4: 433–442.

McCarthy, M. 2000. "US Doctor Pleads Guilty to Murdering Patients." *The Lancet* 356, no. 9234 (September 16): 1010.

McGaghie, W. C. 1990. "Qualitative Variables in Medical School Admission." *Academic Medicine* 65, no. 3 (March): 145–149.
———. 2002. "Assessing Readiness for Medical Education: Evolution of the Medical College Admission Test." *Journal of the American Medical Association* 288, no. 9 (September 4): 1085–1090.

McGaghie, W. C., S. B. Issenberg, E. R. Petrusa, and R. J. Scalese. 2010. "A Critical Review of Simulation-Based Medical Education Research: 2003–2009." *Medical Education* 44, no. 1 (Jan.): 50–63. DOI: 10.1111/j.1365-2923.2009.03547.x

Mennin, S. P., and S. Kalishman. 1998. "Issues and Strategies for Reform in Medical Education: Lessons from Eight Medical Schools." *Academic Medicine* 73, no. 9 (Suppl): S46–54.

Miles, S. H. 2006. *Oath Betrayed: Torture, Medical Complicity, and the War on Terror*. New York: Random House.

Miles, S. H., L. W. Lane, J. Bickel, R. M. Walker, and C. K. Cassel. 1989. "Medical Ethics Education: Coming of Age." *Academic Medicine* 64, no. 12 (Dec.): 705–714.

Miller, F., and H. Brody. 2001. "The Internal Morality of Medicine: An Evolutionary Perspective." *Journal of Medicine and Philosophy* 26, no. 6 (Dec.): 581–599.

MSMW. 1982. "Cheating in Medical School." *The Western Journal of Medicine* 136, no. 2: 145.

Muller, S. 1984. "Physicians for the Twenty-First Century. Report of the Project Panel on the General Professional Education of the Physician and College Preparation for Medicine." *Journal of Medical Education* 59, no. 11 (Pt. 2; Nov.): 1–208.

Murden, R., G. M. Galloway, J. C. Reid, and J. M. Colwill. 1978. "Academic and Personal Predictors of Clinical Success in Medical School." *Journal of Medical Education* 53, no. 9 (Sept.): 711–719.

Mutha, S., J. Takayama, and E. O'Neil. 1997. "Insights into Medical Students' Career Choices based on Third- and Fourth-Year Students' Focus-Group Discussions." *Academic Medicine* 72, no. 7 (July): 635–640.

Nelson, M. S., and M. Eliastam. 1991. "Role-Playing for Teaching Ethics in Emergency Medicine." *American Journal of Emergency Medicine* 9, no. 4 (July): 370–374. DOI: 10.1016/0735-6757(91)90061-n.

Newton, B. W., L. Barber, J. Clardy, E. Cleveland, and P. O'Sullivan. 2008. "Is There Hardening of the Heart during Medical School?" *Academic Medicine* 83, no. 3 (March): 244–249. DOI: 10.1097/ACM.0b013e3181637837. Available at http://journals.lww.com/academicmedicine/fulltext/2008/03000/Is_There_Hardening_of_the_Hear t_During_Medical.6.aspx.

Nussbaum, M. C. 1990. *Love's Knowledge: Essays on Philosophy and Literature*. Oxford: Oxford University Press.

———. 2001. *Upheavals of Thought: The Intelligence of Emotions*. Cambridge: Cambridge University Press.

O'Neill, O. 1987. "Abstraction, Idealization and Ideology in Ethics." *Royal Institute of Philosophy Supplement* 22 (September): 55–69. DOI: 10.1017/S0957042X00003667.

O'Reilly, K. 2009. "TV Doctors' Flaws Become Bioethics Teaching Moments." *American Medical News*, 26 January. Originally accessed in April 2009 at http://www.ama-assn.org/amednews/2009/02/26/prl20126.htm (site discontinued). Archived at https://web.archive.org/web/20090131062451/http://www.ama-assn.org/amednews/2009/01/26/prl20126.htm.

Oakley, J., and D. Cocking. 2001. *Virtue Ethics and Professional Roles*. Cambridge: Cambridge University Press.

Osler, W. 1907. "The Reserves of Life." *St. Mary's Hospital Gazette* 13: 95–98.

———. 1932. *Aequanimitas*. Philadelphia: Blakiston Co.

Overby, P. 2005. "The Moral Education of Doctors." *The New Atlantis*, no. 10 (Fall): 17–26.

Papadakis, M. A., G. K. Arnold, L. L. Blank, E. S. Holmboe, and R. S. Lipner. 2008. "Performance During Internal Medicine Residency Training and Subsequent Disciplinary Action by State Licensing Boards." *Annals of Internal Medicine* 148, no.11 (June 3): 869–876.

Papadakis, M. A., C. S. Hodgson, A. Teherani, and N. D. Kohatsu. 2004. "Unprofessional Behavior in Medical School Is Associated with Subsequent Disciplinary Action by a State Medical Board." *Academic Medicine* 79, no. 3 (March): 244–249.

Papadakis, M. A., H. Loeser, and K. Healy. 2001. "Early Detection and Evaluation of Professionalism Deficiencies in Medical Students: One School's Approach." *Academic Medicine* 76, no. 11 (Nov.): 1100–1106.

Papadakis, M. A., A. Teherani, and M. A. Banach, et al. 2005. "Disciplinary Action by Medical Boards and Prior Behavior in Medical School." *New England Journal of Medicine* 353, no. 25 (Dec. 22): 2673–2682. DOI: 10.1056/NEJMsa052596.

Parker, M. 1995. "Autonomy, Problem-Based Learning, and the Teaching of Medical Ethics." *Journal of Medical Ethics* 21, no. 5 (Oct.): 305–310.

Pascoe, J. M., M. Cox, L. O. Lewin, M. D. Weiss, and K. L. Pye. 2004. "Report on Undergraduate Medical Education for the 21st Century (UME-21): A National Medical Education Project." *Family Medicine* 36, Suppl: S2–S150.

Peabody, F. W. 1927. "The Care of the Patient." *Journal of the American Medical Association* 88, no. 12: 877–882. DOI: 10.1001/jama.1927.02680380001001.

Pellegrino, E. D. 1969. "The Necessity, Promise and Dangers of Human Experimentation." In *Experiments with Man*, 31–56. World Council Studies 6. New York: World Council of Churches, Geneva, and Friendship Press.

———. 1974. "Educating the Humanist Physician: An Ancient Ideal Reconsidered." *Journal of the American Medical Association* 227, no. 11: 1288–1294. DOI: 10.1001/jama.1974.03230240046024.

———. 1979. *Humanism and the Physician*. Knoxville: The University of Tennessee Press.

———. 1986. "Rationing Health Care: The Ethics of Medical Gatekeeping." *Journal of Contemporary Health Law and Policy* 2, no. 1: 23–45.

———. 1989. "Teaching Medical Ethics: Some Persistent Questions and Some Responses." *Academic Medicine* 64, no. 12 (Dec): 701–703.

————. 1992. "Doctors Must Not Kill." *Journal of Clinical Ethics* 3, no. 2 (Summer): 95–102.

————. 1998. "What the Philosophy of Medicine Is." *Theoretical Medicine and Bioethics* 19: 315–336.

————. 1999. "The Goals and Ends of Medicine: How Are They to be Defined?" In *The Goals of Medicine: The Forgotten Issues in Health Care Reform*, edited by M. Hanson and D. Callahan, D. Washington DC: Georgetown University Press.

————. 2001a. "The Internal Morality of Clinical Medicine: A Paradigm for the Ethics of the Helping and Healing Professions." *Journal of Medicine and Philosophy* 26, no. 6: 559–579. DOI: 10.1076/jmep.26.6.559.2998.

————. 2001b. "Philosophy of Medicine: Should It Be Teleologically or Socially Construed?" *Kennedy Institute of Ethics Journal* 11, no. 2: 169–180.

————. 2002a. "Medical Commencement Oaths: Shards of a Fractured Myth, or Seeds of Hope against a Dispiriting Future?" *Medical Journal of Australia* 176, no. 3 (Feb.4): 99.

————. 2002b. "Professionalism, Profession and the Virtues of the Good Physician." *Mount Sinai Journal of Medicine* 69, no. 6 (Nov.): 378–384.

————. 2005a. "Some Things Ought Never Be Done: Moral Absolutes in Clinical Ethics." *Theoretical Medical and Bioethics* 26, no. 6: 469–486.

————. 2005b. "The 'Telos' of Medicine and the Good of the Patient." In *Clinical Bioethics: A Search for the Foundations*, edited by Corrado Viafora, 21–32. New York: Springer-Verlag.

————. 2006. "Toward a Reconstruction of Medical Morality." *American Journal of Bioethics* 6, no. 2: 65–71.

Pellegrino, E. D., R. J. Hart, Jr., S. R. Henderson, S. E. Loef, and G. Edwards. 1985. "Relevance and Utility of Courses in Medical Ethics: A Survey of Physicians' Perceptions." *Journal of the American Medical Association* 253, no. 1 (Jan. 4): 49–53.

Pellegrino, E. D., and D. C. Thomasma. 1981. *A Philosophical Basis of Medical Practice*. New York: Oxford University Press.

Pellegrino, E. D., and D. C. Thomasma. 1993. *The Virtues in Medical Practice. Oxford: Oxford University Press*.

Pence, G. 1983. "Can Compassion Be Taught?" *Journal of Medical Ethics* 9, no. 4 (Dec.): 189–191.

Percival, T. 1803. *Medical Ethics*. Manchester: S. Russell.

Pfifferling, J. H. 1980. *The Impaired Physician*: An Overview. Chapel Hill, NC: Health Sciences Consortium.

————. 1984. "Physicians for the Twenty-First Century: Report of the Project Panel on the General Professional Education of the Physician and College Preparation for Medicine." *Journal of Medical Education* 59 (11 pt. 2): 1–208.

Pickering, G. W. 1956. "The Purpose of Medical Education." *British Medical Journal* 2, no. 4985: 113–116. DOI: 10.1136/bmj.2.4985.113.

Pindar. 1924. *The Odes of Pythiae, including the Principal Fragments*. Introduced and translated by Sir John Sandys. New York: Putnam.

Plato. 1942. *The Republic*. Translated by Francis Macdonald Cornford, Oxford: Oxford University Press.

Plato. 2013. *Dialogues of Plato*. Enriched Classics edition. New York: Simon and Schuster.

Puschmann, T. 1966. *A History of Medical Education*. New York: Hafner Publishing Co.

Quill, T. E. 1991. "Death and Dignity. A Case of Individualized Decision Making." *New England Journal of Medicine* 324, no. 10 (Mar. 7): 691–694. DOI: 10.1056/NEJM199103073241010.

Rao, K. N. 1961. "Trends in Medical Education in the World." *Journal of Medical Education* 36, no. 9 (Sep.): 1233–1244.

Reed, R., and D. Evans. 1987. "The Deprofessionalization of Medicine. Causes, Effects, and Responses." *Journal of the American Medical Association* 258, no. 22 (Dec. 11): 3279–3282.

Reiter, H. I., and K. W. Eva. 2005. "Reflecting the Relative Values of Community, Faculty and Students in the Admissions Tools of Medical School." *Teaching and Learning in Medicine* 17, no. 1 (Winter): 4–8.

Reuler, J., and D. Nardone. 1994. "Role Modeling in Medical Education." *Western Journal of Medicine* 160, no. 4 (April): 335–337.

Reynolds, P. 1994. "Reaffirming Professionalism Through the Education Community." *Annals of Internal Medicine* 120, no. 7 (Apr. 1): 609–614.

Rogers, A. 1996. *Teaching Adults.* Buckingham/Philadelphia: Open University Press.

Romanelli, F., J. Cain, and K. M. Smith. 2006. "Emotional Intelligence as a Predictor of Academic and/or Professional Success." *American Journal of Pharmaceutical Education* 70, no. 3 (June 15): 69. DOI: 10.5688/aj700369.

Rosenberg, D. A., and H. K. Silver. 1984. "Medical Student Abuse. An Unnecessary and Preventable Cause of Stress." *Journal of the American Medical Association* 251, no. 6 (Feb. 10): 739–742. DOI: 10.1001/jama.251.6.739.

Ryle, G. 1958. "On Forgetting the Difference Between Right and Wrong." In *Essays in Moral Philosophy*, edited by A. I. Melden, 147–159. Seattle: University of Washington Press.

Salvatori, P. 2001. "Reliability and Validity of Admissions Tools Used to Select Students for the Health Professions." *Advances in Health Sciences Education* 6, no. 2: 159–175.

Schein, E. H. 1983. "The Role of the Founder in Creating Organizational Culture." *Organizational Dynamics*, 12, no. 1 (Summer): 13–28.

Sheehan, K. H., D. V. Sheehan, K. White, A. Leibowitz, and D. C. Baldwin, Jr. 1990. "A Pilot Study of Medical Student 'Abuse'. Student Perceptions of Mistreatment and Misconduct in Medical School." *Journal of American Medical Association* 263, no. 4 (Jan. 26): 533–537.

Shelton, W. 1999. "Can Virtue Be Taught?" *Academic Medicine* 74, no. 6 (June): 671–674.

Shryock, R. H. 1947. *The Development of Modern Medicine: An Interpretation of the Social and Scientific Factors Involved.* New York: Alfred A. Knopf Inc.

Silver, H. K. 1982. "Medical Students and Medical School." *Journal of the American Medical Association* 247, no. 3 (Jan. 15): 309–310.

Slote, M. 2010. *Moral Sentimentalism.* New York: Oxford University Press.
———. 2012. *Education and Human Values: Reconciling Talent with an Ethics of Care.* New York/Abingdon: Routledge.

Smith, R. 2000. "Cheating at Medical School." *British Medical Journal* 321, no. 7258: 398. DOI: 10.1136/bmj.321.7258.398.

Sockett, H. 1976. *Designing the Curriculum.* London, Open Books.

Sokol, D. 2008. "The Essence of Medicine." *British Medical Journal*, vol. 336, no. 7654 (May 24): 1163. DOI: 10.1136/bmj.39583.748727.94.

Solomon, D. 1988. "Internal Objections to Virtue Ethics." *Midwest Studies in Philosophy* 13, no. 1: 428–441.

Spiro, H. 2006. "To the Editor." *Journal of the American Medical Association* 295, no. 9: 997.

Spiro, H., and P. W. Norton. 2003. "Dean Milton C. Winternitz at Yale." *Perspectives in Biology and Medicine* 46, no. 3 (Summer): 403–412.

Starfield, B. 2000. "Is US Health Really the Best in the World?" *Journal of the American Medical Association* 284, no. 4 (July 26): 483–485. DOI: 10.1001/jama.284.4.483.

Steinbrook, R. 2002. "Protecting Research Subjects: The Crisis at Johns Hopkins." *New England Journal of Medicine* 346, no. 9 (Feb. 28): 716–720.

Stenhouse, L. 1975. *An Introduction to Curriculum Research and Development*. London: Heinemann.

Stern, C., and M. Papadakis. 2006. "The Developing Physician – Becoming a Professional." *New England Journal of Medicine* 355, no. 17: 1794–1799.

Steward, J. B. 1999. *Blind Eye: How the Medical Establishment Let a Doctor Get Away with Murder*. New York: Simon & Schuster.

Stocker, N. 1976. "The Schizophrenia of Modern Theories." *The Journal of Philosophy* 73, no. 14: 453–466. DOI: 10.2307/2025782.

Sugarman, J., and D. Sulmasy. 2010. *Methods in Medical Ethics*. Washington DC: Georgetown University Press.

Sulmasy, D. 2006. *The Rebirth of the Clinic: An Introduction to Spirituality in Healthcare*. Washington DC: Georgetown University Press.

Swick, H. M. 2000. "Toward a Normative Definition of Medical Professionalism." *Academic Medicine* 75, no. 6: 612–616.

Swick, H. M., P. Szenas, D. Danoff, and M. E. Whitcomb. 1999. "Teaching Professionalism in Undergraduate Medical Education."*Journal of the American Medical Association* 282, no. 9 (Sept. 1): 830–832.

Tamblyn, R., M. Abrahamowicz, D. Dauphinee, et al. 2007. "Physician Scores on a National Clinical Skills Examination as Predictors of Complaints to Medical Regulatory Authorities." *Journal of the American Medical Association* 298, no. 9 (Sept. 5): 993–1001.

Taylor, B. C. 1997. "Nuclear Pictures and Metapictures." *American Literary History* vol. 9, no. 3 (Autumn): 567–597.

Testerman, J. K., K. R. Morton, L. K. Loo, J. S. Worthley, and H. H. Lamberton. 1996. "The Natural History of Cynicism in Physicians." *Academic Medicine* 71, 10 suppl. (Oct.): S43–45.

Tolkin, L., and S. Glick. 2007. "Ethical Behavioral Standards of Medical Students on Examinations and Studies." *Harefuah* 146, no. 6 (June): 429–434.

Tolstoy, L. 1967. *Great Short Works of Leo Tolstoy*. Translated by Louise and Aylmer Maude. New York: Harper and Row.

Tonchev, A. B., T. Yamashima, L. Zhao, H. J. Okano, and H. Okano. 2003. "Proliferation of Neural and Neuronal Progenitors after Global Brain Ischemia in Young Adult Macaque Monkeys." *Molecular Cell Neuroscience* 23, no. 2: 292–301.

Tysinger, J.W, L. K. Klonis, J. Z. Sadler, and J. M. Wagner. 1997. "Teaching Ethics Using Small-Group, Problem-Based Learning." *Journal of Medical Ethics* 23, no. 5: 315–318.

UNESCO. 2010. *Teaching and Learning for a Sustainable Future*. http://www.unesco.org/education/tlsf/.

Urmson, J. O. 1958. "Saints and heroes." In *Essays in Moral Philosophy*, edited by A. I. Welden, 198–216. Seattle: University of Washington Press.

Veatch, R. M. 2001. "The Impossibility of a Morality Internal to Medicine." *Journal of Medicine and Philosophy* 26, no. 6: 621–642.

Wagner, P. J. 2006. "Does High EI (Emotional Intelligence) Make Better Doctors?" *Virtual Mentor* 8, no. 7: 477–479. DOI: 10.1001/virtualmentor.2006.8.7.oped2-0607.

Walker, F. 2005. "Cultivating Simple Virtues in Medicine." *Neurology* 65, No. 10: 1678–1680. DOI: 10.1212/01.wnl.0000185110.10041.7c.

Wear, D. 1998.) "On White Coats and Professional Development: The Formal and the Hidden Curricula." *Annals of Internal Medicine* 129, no. 9 (Nov. 1): 734–737.

Wear, D., and J. Zarconi. 2008. "Can Compassion Be Taught? Let's Ask Our Students." *Journal of General Internal Medicine* 23, no. 7 (July): 948–953.

Weingartner, R. H. 1980. "Selecting for Medical School." *Journal of Medical Education*, vol. 55, no. 11: 922–927.

Weinstein, H. M. 1983. "A Committee on Well-Being of Medical Students and House Staff." *Journal of Medical Education* 58, no. 5 (May): 373–381.

Wensing, M., H. P. Jung, J. Mainz, F. Olesen, and R. Grol. 1998. "A Systematic Review of the Literature on Patient Priorities for General Practice Care. Part 1: Description of the Research Domain." *Social Science Medicine* 47, no. 10 (Nov.): 1573–1588.

Wildes, K. W. 2001. "The Crisis of Medicine: Philosophy and the Social Construction of Medicine." *Kennedy Institute of Ethics Journal* 11, no. 1 (March): 71–86.

Wilson, L. O. 2005. *Curriculum Index*. Originally accessed in January 2010 at http://www. uwsp.edu/Education/lwilson/curric/curtyp.htm (site discontinued). Available at "The Second Principle. The work of Leslie Owen Wilson, Ed. D." https://thesecondprinciple.com/ instructional-design/.

Wolf, T. M., P. M. Balson, J.M. Faucett, and H. M. Randall. 1989. "A Retrospective Study of Attitude Change During Medical Education." *Medical Education* 23, no. 1: 19–23.

Wright, S. 1996. "Examining What Residents Look for in Their Role Models." *Academic Medicine* 71, no. 3 (March): 290–292.

Wright, S., and J. A. Carrese. 2002. "Excellence in Role Modelling: Insight and Perspectives from the Pros." *Canadian Medical Association Journal* 167, no. 6 (Sep. 17): 638–643.

Wright, S. M., D. E. Kern, K. Kolodner, D. M. Howard, and F. L. Brancati. 1998. "Attributes of Excellent Attending-Physician Role Models." *New England Journal of Medicine* 339, no. 27 (Dec. 31): 1986–1993.

Wright, S., A. Wong, and C. Newill. 1997. "The Impact of Role Models on Medical Students", *Journal of General Internal Medicine* 12, no. 1: 53–56. DOI: 10.1046/j.1525-1497.1997.12109.x.

Wynia, M. K., S. R. Latham, A. C. Kao, J. W. Berg, and L. L. Emanuel. 1999. "Medical Professionalism in Society." *New England Journal of Medicine* 341: 1612–1616. DOI: 10.1056/NEJM199911183412112.

Yale University School of Medicine. 2016. *Mission Statement and School Wide Objectives*. https://medicine.yale.edu/education/ppgg/images/Mission%20Statement_2016_tcm63-283674.pdf.

Young, Y. 1987. "Faculty Development and the Concept of 'Profession'." *Academe* 73, no. 3 (May-June): 12–14.

Zastowny, T. R., W. C. Stratmann, E. H. Adams, and M. L. Fox. 1995. "Patient Satisfaction and

Experience with Health Services and Quality of Care." *Quality Management in Health Care* 3, no. 3 (spring): 50–61.

Zezima, K. 2009. "Experiencing Life, Briefly, Inside a Nursing Home." *New York Times*, August 23, accessed 19 March 2010, https://www.nytimes.com/2009/08/24/health/24nursing.html.

Zhang, R. L., Z. G. Zhang, and M. Chopp. 2005. "Neurogenesis in the Adult Ischemic Brain: Generation, Migration, Survival, and Restorative Therapy." *Neuroscientist* 11, no. 5: 408–416.